Psychiatric and Behavioral Emergencies

Editors

EILEEN F. BAKER
CATHERINE A. MARCO

EMERGENCY MEDICINE CLINICS OF NORTH AMERICA

www.emed.theclinics.com

Consulting Editor
AMAL MATTU

February 2024 • Volume 42 • Number 1

ELSEVIER

1600 John F. Kennedy Boulevard ● Suite 1800 ● Philadelphia, Pennsylvania, 19103-2899

http://www.theclinics.com

EMERGENCY MEDICINE CLINICS OF NORTH AMERICA Volume 42, Number 1
February 2024 ISSN 0733-8627, ISBN-13: 978-0-443-18236-5

Editor: Joanna Gascoine
Developmental Editor: Varun Gopal

Emergency Medicine Clinics of North America (ISSN 0733-8627) is published quarterly by Elsevier Inc., 360 Park Avenue South, New York, NY, 10010-1710. Months of issue are February, May, August, and November. Business and Editorial Offices: 1600 John F. Kennedy Boulevard, Suite 1800, Philadelphia, PA 19103-2899. Customer Service Office: 6277 Sea Harbor Drive, Orlando, FL 32887-4800. Periodicals postage paid at New York, NY, and additional mailing offices. Subscription prices are $100.00 per year (US students), $388.00 per year (US individuals), $220.00 per year (international students), $505.00 per year (international individuals), $100.00 per year (Canadian students), $463.00 per year (Canadian individuals). For institutional access pricing please contact Customer Service via the contact information below. International air speed delivery is included in all *Clinics'* subscription prices. All prices are subject to change without notice. **POSTMASTER:** Send address changes to *Emergency Medicine Clinics of North America*, Elsevier Periodicals Customer Service, 11830 Westline Industrial Drive, St. Louis, MO 63146. Customer Service (orders, claims, online, change of address): Elsevier Periodicals **Customer Service, 11830 Westline Industrial Drive, St. Louis, MO 63146. Tel: 1-800-654-2452 (U.S. and Canada); 314-453-7041 (outside U.S. and Canada). Fax: 314-453-5170. E-mail: journalscustomerservice-usa@elsevier.com (for print support); journalsonlinesupport-usa@elsevier.com (for online support).**

Reprints. For copies of 100 or more of articles in this publication, please contact the Commercial Reprints Department, Elsevier Inc., 360 Park Avenue South, New York, NY 10010-1710. Tel.: 212-633-3874; Fax: 212-633-3820; E-mail: reprints@elsevier.com.

Emergency Medicine Clinics of North America is covered in *MEDLINE/PubMed (Index Medicus), Current Contents/Clinical Medicine, EMBASE/Excerpta Medica, BIOSIS, SciSearch, CINAHL, ISI/BIOMED,* and *Research Alert.*

Contributors

CONSULTING EDITOR

AMAL MATTU, MD
Professor and Vice Chair of Academic Affairs, Department of Emergency Medicine, University of Maryland School of Medicine, Baltimore, Maryland, USA

EDITORS

EILEEN F. BAKER, MD, PhD, FACEP
Emergency Physician Riverwood Emergency Services, Inc, Perrysburg, Ohio, USA

CATHERINE A. MARCO, MD, FACEP
Professor, Department of Emergency Medicine, Penn State Health Milton S. Hershey Medical Center, Hershey, Pennsylvania, USA

AUTHORS

INA BECKER, MD, PhD
Assistant Professor of Psychiatry, Columbia University, Vagelos College of Physicians and Surgeon, New York, New York, USA

ADAM BERNSTEIN, MD
Resident in Adult Psychiatry, Creedmoor Psychiatric Center, New York State Office of Mental Health, Queens, New York, USA

JAY M. BRENNER, MD
Professor of Emergency Medicine, SUNY–Upstate Medical University, Syracuse, New York, USA

SAMANTHA CHAO, MD, HEC-C
House Officer, Department of Emergency Medicine, University of Michigan, Ann Arbor, Michigan, USA

MONICA CORSETTI, MD
Emergency Medicine Physician, Penn State Health Holy Spirit Medical Center, Camp Hill, Pennsylvania, USA

JAMES FERRY, DO
Emergency Medicine Physician, Department of Emergency Medicine, Geisinger, Danville, Pennsylvania, USA

MICHELLE A. FISCHER, MD, MPH
Associate Professor of Emergency Medicine, Residency Program Director, Department of Emergency Medicine, Penn State Health Milton S. Hershey Medical Center, Penn State College of Medicine, Hershey, Pennsylvania, USA

DIANE L. GORGAS, MD
Professor, Vice Chair of Academic Affairs, Department of Emergency Medicine, Executive Director, Health Sciences Center for Global Health, The Ohio State University, Columbus, Ohio, USA

PURVA GROVER, MD, MBA
Clinical Associate Professor, Emergency Medicine, CWRU, Cleveland Clinic, Mayfield Heights, Ohio, USA

ARTUN K. KADASTER, BS
Department of Anesthesia, Mayo Clinic, Rochester, Minnesota, USA

EMILY ANNE KIERNAN, DO
Assistant Professor, Department of Emergency Medicine, Emory University School of Medicine, Georgia Poison Center, Atlanta, Georgia, USA

CHADD K. KRAUS, DO, DrPH, CME, FACEP
Vice Chair, Research, Department of Emergency and Hospital Medicine, Lehigh Valley Health Network, Allentown, Pennsylvania, USA; Professor, University of South Florida Morsani College of Medicine

MANYA KUMAR, MBBS
Vardhman Mahavir Medical College, Safdarjung Hospital, New Delhi, Delhi, India

RYAN E. LAWRENCE, MD
Director, Comprehensive Psychiatric Emergency Program, Associate Professor of Psychiatry at CUMC, Columbia University Irving Medical Center, NewYork-Presbyterian Hospital, New York, New York, USA

NICOLE MCCOIN, MD
Chair, Department of Emergency Medicine, Ochsner Medical Center, New Orleans, Louisiana, USA

JILLIAN L. MCGRATH, MD
Associate Professor Clinical, Department of Emergency Medicine, The Ohio State University Wexner Medical Center, Columbus, Ohio, USA

BRIAN PATRICK MURRAY, DO
Assistant Professor, Department of Emergency Medicine, Wright State Boonshoft School of Medicine, Dayton, Ohio, USA

MAEGAN S. REYNOLDS, MD
Assistant Professor Clinical, Department of Emergency Medicine and Pediatrics, The Ohio State University Wexner Medical Center, Nationwide Children's Hospital, Division of Emergency Medicine, Department of Emergency Medicine, Columbus, Ohio, USA

THOMAS E. ROBEY, MD, PhD
Assistant Professor of Emergency Medicine, Elson S. Floyd College of Medicine, Washington State University, Providence Regional Medical Center Everett, Everett, Washington, USA

STEPHEN SANDELICH, MD
Attending Physician, Pediatric Emergency Medicine, Assistant Professor, Emergency Medicine and Pediatrics, Penn State Health Milton S. Hershey Medical Center, Hershey, Pennsylvania, USA

MARKAYLE R. SCHEARS, MPH
University of Wisconsin-Madison School of Medicine and Public Health, Madison, Wisconsin, USA

RAQUEL M. SCHEARS, MD, MPH, MBA, FACEP
Professor, University of Central Florida, Orlando, Florida, USA

BRIAN SPRINGER, MD, FACEP
Professor and Vice Chair, Director, Division of Tactical Emergency Medicine, Department of Emergency Medicine, Wright State University, Dayton, Ohio, USA

KAITLYN R. SWIMMER, MD
Pediatric Resident, Department of Pediatrics, Penn State Health Milton S. Hershey Medical Center, Hershey, Pennsylvania, USA

CARMEN WOLFE, MD
Physician, Department of Emergency Medicine, TriStar Skyline Medical Center, Nashville, Tennessee, USA

Contents

A quality clinical interview helps establish a good collaborative relationship with the patient. This is especially important when emergency physicians conduct a psychiatric interview. Familiarity with interview techniques, empathic listening, and observation of nonverbal cues, behavior, and appearance enhance diagnostic excellence.

The acutely agitated patient should be managed in a step-wise fashion, beginning with non-coercive de-escalation strategies and moving on to pharmacologic interventions and physical restraints as necessary. Face-to-face examination, monitoring, and documentation by the physician are essential. The emergency physician should be familiar with multiple pharmaceutical options, tailored to the individual patient. Use of ketamine, benzodiazepines and antipsychotics should be considered. Patient autonomy, safety, and medical well-being are paramount.

Patients frequently present to the emergency department (ED) with acute suicidal and homicidal thoughts. These patients require timely evaluation, with determination of disposition by either voluntary or involuntary hospitalization or discharge with appropriate outpatient follow-up. Safety concerns should be prioritized for patients as well as ED staff. Patient dignity and autonomy should be respected throughout the process.

Hyperactive delirium with severe agitation is a clinical syndrome of altered mental status, psychomotor agitation, and a hyperadrenergic state. The underlying pathophysiology is variable and often results from sympathomimetic abuse, psychiatric disease, sedative-hypnotic withdrawal, and metabolic derangement. Patients can go from a combative state to periarrest with little warning. Safety of the patient and of the medical providers is paramount and the emergency department should be prepared to manage these patients with adequate staffing, restraints, and pharmacologic sedatives. Treatment with benzodiazepines, antipsychotics, or ketamine is recommended, followed by airway protection, supportive measures, and cooling of hyperthermia.

Depressive disorders encompass a spectrum of diagnoses and are more common in women and transgender individuals. Diagnosis involves thorough history-taking and exclusion of underlying medical disorders. The emergency physician should assess the risk of self-harm and consider environmental and social factors prior to disposition.

Affective disorders affect the way that people think and feel and are classified into unipolar disorders and bipolar disorders. Bipolar disorders represent a spectrum of these chronic mental health illnesses. Patients with bipolar disorder have high recurrence of acute symptoms, and on average spend 20% of their life in exacerbations characterized by mania, depression, or psychosis. Given the increased morbidity and mortality associated with bipolar disorders, it is imperative that the emergency physician remain vigilant when these patients seek emergency care.

Caring for patients with personality disorders and traits presents unique challenges for physicians and other providers. The Diagnostic and Statistical Manual of Mental Disorders, Fifth Edition, recognizes 10 personality disorders, which are organized into 3 clusters (A, B, and C) based on shared diagnostic features. Personality disorders or traits create difficulty in clinical and interpersonal interactions, promoting missed diagnosis or underdiagnosis, nonadherence to medical recommendations, or other dangerous outcomes. It is important to recognize patients with potential personality disorders and understand strategies to achieve optimal patient interactions and best possible medical outcomes.

Geriatric patients, those 65 years of age and older, often experience psychiatric symptoms or changes in mentation as a manifestation of an organic illness. It is crucial to recognize and treat delirium in these patients as it is often under-recognized and associated with significant morbidity. Iatrogenic causes of altered mentation or delirium due to medication adverse reactions are common. Treatment of the underlying cause, creating an environment conducive to orientation, and minimizing agitation and discomfort are first-line interventions. Antipsychotics are first-line pharmacologic interventions if needed to preserve patient safety.

Pediatric psychiatric emergencies account for 15% of emergency department visits and are on the rise. Psychiatric diagnoses in the pediatric population are difficult to make, due to their variable presentation, but early diagnosis and treatment improve clinical outcome. Medical reasons for the patient's presentation should be explored. Both physical and emotional safety must be ensured. A multidisciplinary approach, utilizing local primary care and psychiatric resources, is recommended.

EMERGENCY MEDICINE
CLINICS OF NORTH AMERICA

SERIES OF RELATED INTEREST

Critical Care Clinics
https://www.criticalcare.theclinics.com/
Cardiology Clinics
https://www.cardiology.theclinics.com/

THE CLINICS ARE NOW AVAILABLE ONLINE!
Access your subscription at:
www.theclinics.com

EMERGENCY MEDICINE
CLINICS OF NORTH AMERICA

FORTHCOMING ISSUES

May 2025
Infectious Disease Emergencies
Christopher M. Colbert, Rachel E. Bridwell,
and Michael Pulia, Editors

August 2024
Environmental and Wilderness Medicine
Cheyenne Falat and Stephanie Lareau,
Editors

November 2024
Clinical Ultrasound in the Emergency
Department
Michael Gottlieb and Alexis Salerno,
Editors

RECENT ISSUES

November 2022
Endocrine and Metabolic Emergencies
Tiffany M. Abramson and Bennett A. Myers,
Editors

August 2022
Cardiac Arrest
William Brady, Amandeep Singh,
Editors

May 2022
Updates in Obstetrics and Gynecology
Emergencies
Sreeja Natesan, Joelle Borhart, and Sophia Lin, Editors

SERIES OF RELATED INTEREST

Cardiology Clinics
http://www.cardiology.theclinics.com
Heart Failure Clinics
http://www.heartfailure.theclinics.com

THE CLINICS ARE NOW AVAILABLE ONLINE!
Access your subscription at:
www.theclinics.com

Foreword

Psychiatric and Behavioral Emergencies

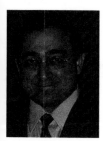

Amal Mattu, MD
Editor

"Life is not easy." These were the words of wisdom that one of my mentors in residency would often say to us as an explanation for the difficulties that many of our patients faced. These difficulties often led to ED visits for psychiatric and behavioral emergencies. That was back in the 1990s, and it seems that life has just become progressively more complicated since then. The result, it seems, is that we see more behavioral health emergencies in the ED than ever before. Stress and anxiety disorder, depression, and bipolar disorder are being diagnosed more than ever before. Whether this phenomenon can be attributed to the recent COVID-19 pandemic and social isolation, to problems in society such as racism, or other social issues, or attributed to improvements in screening and diagnosing behavior health conditions, we in emergency medicine need to understand these conditions more than ever before.

In this issue of *Emergency Medicine Clinics of North America*, two experts in the field of psychiatric and behavioral emergencies have stepped up to teach us what we need to know to optimally recognize and treat these patients. Guest editors Drs Eileen Baker and Catherine Marco have assembled an outstanding group of educators and writers to inform us of best practices in an assortment of psychiatric and behavioral disorders. The first topic they address is perhaps the most important—how to conduct a cost-effective initial evaluation that helps to detect overt or subtle psychiatric illness. The authors also address core topics, such as depression and suicidal thoughts, bipolar disorder, schizophrenia, eating disorders, and personality disorders. Two articles are devoted to substance abuse, very appropriate given the tremendous association between illicit drugs and behavior disorders. Agitated delirium is addressed, as are the special populations of elderly and pediatric patients. Two final articles are provided that address "difficult patients" and also legal and ethical considerations.

Emerg Med Clin N Am 42 (2024) xiii–xiv
https://doi.org/10.1016/j.emc.2023.09.002
0733-8627/24/© 2023 Published by Elsevier Inc.

emed.theclinics.com

In total, this issue of *Emergency Medicine Clinics of North America* represents an outstanding resource for emergency physicians and other acute care providers, especially in a time when it seems that psychiatric and behavioral emergencies are increasing in ED practice. Congratulations to the authors and editors for an invaluable contribution to our ED practice!

Amal Mattu, MD
Department of Emergency Medicine
University of Maryland School of Medicine
Baltimore, MD, USA

E-mail address:
amattu@som.umaryland.edu

Preface

Essentials of Psychiatric and Behavioral Emergencies

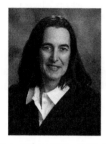
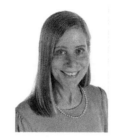

Eileen F. Baker, MD, PhD, FACEP   Catherine A. Marco, MD, FACEP

Editors

Psychiatric emergencies are increasingly common in the practice of Emergency Medicine. A comprehensive knowledge of psychiatric conditions, including both acute and chronic conditions, is essential to the emergency department management of these conditions. This issue of *Emergency Medicine Clinics of North America* on psychiatric emergencies opens with a description of the psychiatric interview and then focuses on several crucial topics for emergency physicians (management of the agitated patient, suicidal or homicidal symptoms, hyperactive delirium with severe agitation, substance use disorder, and physiologic effects of substance use). It then moves to more classic psychiatric illnesses, including schizophrenia, depression, bipolar disorder, and personality disorders. The final third of the issue explores a range of topics, from geriatric to pediatric emergencies, eating disorders, and malingering, concluding with a study of legal and ethical issues in psychiatric emergencies.

We appreciate the authors' expertise, creating what we believe is a concise, yet thorough exploration of essential topics in psychiatric emergency medicine. We are grateful to the editorial staff of *Emergency Medicine Clinics of North America* for their work in crafting this issue. We hope the reader finds this information both informative and practical in its application.

Emerg Med Clin N Am 42 (2024) xv–xvi
https://doi.org/10.1016/j.emc.2023.09.001
0733-8627/24/© 2023 Published by Elsevier Inc.

Conflict of interest/disclosures: The authors have no conflicts to disclose.

Eileen F. Baker, MD, PhD, FACEP
Riverwood Emergency Services, Inc
Perrysburg, OH, USA

Catherine A. Marco, MD, FACEP
Department of Emergency Medicine
Penn State Health–
Milton S. Hershey Medical Center
Hershey, PA, USA

E-mail addresses:
uhemsdoc@earthlink.net (E.F. Baker)
cmarco2@aol.com (C.A. Marco)

The Emergency Psychiatric Interview

Ina Becker, MD, PhD

KEYWORDS

- Diagnostic interview • Emergency psychiatric interview • Talking to patients
- Talking to psychiatric patients • The compassionate interview
- The noncooperative patient

KEY POINTS

- A good initial interview is the beginning of most medical encounters; it establishes a collaborative relationship with the patient.
- Many emergency departments rely on emergency physicians to see psychiatric patients before expert consultants can be called to assist.
- Basic facility with the techniques of interviewing and components of the interview will enhance diagnostic excellence for all patients.
- Behavioral observation (nonverbal interview) still yields important information toward diagnosis and is the first step toward treatment.

INTRODUCTION

Emergency physicians are often the first doctor to encounter a patient who is presenting for help. They are tasked with triaging a variety of presenting complaints and illnesses, including psychiatric problems, and are usually in charge of recommending treatments or at least next steps toward diagnosis. In almost all encounters with patients, the interview is the most important instrument in a clinicians' tool kit, regardless if the presenting complaint be medical or psychiatric. A psychiatric interview tends to be much more comprehensive than a medical intake and thus is a good model for practicing general interviewing skills. A good interview includes basic steps toward establishing a relationship between two people, in this case for the purpose of helping the patient with their presenting complaint.

Careful listening during the interview will also reveal much relevant emotional content that may help or hinder the treatment process. Many patients are afraid of doctors in general, unsure about what is happening to them or their bodies. Others are highly anxious in this situation, which may disrupt their ability to explain their symptoms.

No financial conflicts.
Columbia University, Vagelos College of Physicians and Surgeon, CUMC, CPEP, Room 130, 622 West 168 Street, New York, NY 10032, USA
E-mail address: ib58@cumc.columbia.edu

Emerg Med Clin N Am 42 (2024) 1–11
https://doi.org/10.1016/j.emc.2023.06.020
0733-8627/24/© 2023 Elsevier Inc. All rights reserved.

Empathic listening is the most powerful tool in making people feel more comfortable during their examination.

If the treating physician assumes a compassionate stance during the interview, this will have a measurable, positive effect on outcome of treatment.[1,2] A compassionate, collaborative relationship, making validating, compassionate statements about a patient's distress only lengthens a patient encounter by roughly an additional 45 seconds of time.[1]

In addition, great interviewing continues to be a primary skill that physicians can improve over years of study and practice. Understanding the essential structure of the psychiatric interview helps develop listening skills and this in turn will improve diagnostic accuracy.[3] With an emphasis on relating to a person, rather than "a symptom" or "a problem," patients may feel comfortable explaining additional, valuable factors such as stress levels, recent losses, or extent of substance use.

Interview Basics

The psychiatric interview has changed in structure and form over the last 3 decades, because the advent of neuroscience and Diagnostic and Statistical Manual/International Classification of Diseases (DSM/ICD) catalogues of categorization of mental disorders according to descriptive criteria rather than psychodynamic/psychological formulations that see human functioning as being based on the interaction of drives and forces within the person[4–7] In many aspects, this resembles more a general medical interview than the psychodynamic intakes of decades past.

The number of patients presenting to emergency departments with psychiatric complaints has also increased over the last few decades. Today, every emergency physician needs to have familiarity with conducting a psychiatric interview.

The basic structure of any initial patient encounter should contain introductions, discussion of the chief complaint, eliciting details of symptoms/experiences that help lead to diagnosis, and discussion of the presumptive diagnosis and proposed further diagnostic tests and treatment plan. This format is the same for a psychiatric interview. Such an interview consists of three phases.

1. The opening phase: introductions and formation of a treatment alliance. The opening phase of the interview may seem trivial or superficial, like any chat with a stranger but may be most vital for ensuring a collaborative relationship with the patient and compliance with treatment and aftercare. Research has shown that patients are more likely to follow recommendations of a physician who has good bedside manners to whom they can relate on a personal level.
2. Data collection: symptoms, subjective and objective signs of the underlying problem, medical, social, and substance use histories.
3. The closing phase: assessment and formulation and making recommendations for a treatment plan or next steps (admission/discharge with outpatient follow-up, additional tests). Often, a diagnosis can be made after an initial interview, but not always. The interview should always lead to recommendations for next steps to take in the process of helping the patient.

PHASE 1: THE OPENING PHASE

First, we set up the physical environment for the interview. Many emergency departments are open noisy spaces and not conducive to privacy. Effort should be taken to create as much privacy as possible.

And safety first! Before even beginning an interview, the safety of patient and interviewer must be established. Is the patient medically stable for a conversation? Is there a risk of violence or agitation? Is the patient intoxicated or otherwise highly unpredictable? If the answer is yes to any of these questions, the interview should be terminated and consist of observation only, until safety can be established.

During the initial encounter, physicians often will have only very rudimentary information from a triage nurse outlining the patient's reason for presenting for help, and in the case of agitated, intoxicated or otherwise nonverbal patients, even less. The most valuable opening question for any interview is a direct question: "What brings you in today? How can I help you?"

Elements of a complete psychiatric interview include.

- Appearance
- Behavior
- Speech
- Thinking
- Mood/affect
- Hallucinations
- Delusions
- Suicidal/homicidal ideation
- Safety evaluation
- Cognitive examination
- Insight/judgment
- Medical problems/clearance
- Substance use
- Parallel history/family/other sources for history

Chief Complaint and Beginning the Interview: Appearance and Behavior: Introductions

The art of creating a connection with a patient in an area of high acuity and often tremendous time pressure is a learned skill. For many patients, an emergency department (ED) visit constitutes one of the worst days of their lives. People are highly stressed. Most do not know medical terms for their symptoms. They will tell their stories in their own words. Active empathic listening helps the patient feel understood and enhances diagnostic accuracy. It helps establish a collaborative relationship. If a patient perceives the doctor to be kind and compassionate, they tend to be more open about often embarrassing feelings or experiences.

Research has shown that once a patient begins to explain why they are in the ED, they get interrupted after about 23 seconds.[1]

A patient who trusts their physician is more likely to follow recommendations and adhere to recommended treatments.[1] Adopting a compassionate style takes an additional 45 seconds of time on average. It improves outcomes for patients and reduces burnout in medical staff.[1]

The interview begins with observation. When approaching the patient, observe the person's appearance, demeanor, dress, grooming, and psychomotor activity. Does the person's behavior seem normal? Would they stand out in a public setting? Nonverbal communications are 90% of all communication. Does he seem nervous, or does she seem sad, slumped over, or oddly dressed? Does he have odd facial expressions, as if listening to content from inside his head? Does she seem disorganized? Lost? Physical abnormalities? Limp, injuries? Observe their behavior. How is their eye contact? Body language? Level of arousal? Do they demonstrate disinhibition? What is the level of engagement and rapport?

If possible, sit across from the patient and make eye contact. Introduce yourself and your role. A few general comments may be ice breakers and can put the person at ease.

PHASE 2: DATA COLLECTION

Once a connection is established and the chief complaint has been elicited, the interviewer poses a few open questions. Why today? Did the patient come by himself/herself? How would he/she/they like to be addressed? Ask occasional open follow-up questions to clarify information, such as "Do you mean you have been feeling sad and depressed since your mother died? How does that affect your daily life?" Open questions allow for the patient's own thoughts to come through and allow us to learn about their internal process, thoughts, and feeling states.

Begin to elicit associated symptoms, for example, if the person is depressed, do they feel hopeless and helpless, tired, and unmotivated. Do they experience sleep problems, a loss of appetite? Is it difficult to get out of bed? Does (s)he experience suicidal ideation (SI)?

Speech

Speech is the outward presentation of underlying thought content. Is there dysarthria or other speech impediment? Does the speech flow in a normal speed and rhythm? Is it loud or whispered? Is it highly excited or monotonous? Is it monosyllabic or voluminous? Notice any abnormality.

Thinking

Normal thought tends to proceed in a linear, predominantly logical fashion, such as in storytelling. In interviewing a patient, we want to measure the presentation of thought against the typical flow of conversation. How does it vary from this?

Is the thought process logical and linear, goal-oriented and understandable? Or is it very fast, rapid, pressured, like in mania? Or is there barely any thought, such as in thought blocking of psychosis, where patients begin a sentence or utter a single word and are incapable of finishing it and become silent mid-sentence? This is most severe in catatonia, where patients may lose their ability to speak altogether.

In poverty of thought that often accompanies depression, patients seem to think very slowly, have no ideas and can barely express simple issues, and have long speech latency before beginning a new sentence. Speech is often monosyllabic, just a few words.

What is the content of thoughts? What are the subjects? Is there excessive worry, rumination, like in anxiety disorders? Is there perseveration or confabulation, such as in dementia or delirium? Or is the content of a bizarre nature? What is the thought form? Logical or illogical?

Are thought insertion/withdrawal/broadcasting present, such as in some psychoses?

Is the thought process so jumbled that it seems to be word salad? Does it get immediately derailed, in tangential thinking? Is there clanging (repeating the interviewers last words and rhyming it with similar words), or echolalia (repetition of the interviewer's words)? Or is the speech filled with neologisms, non-sensical words?

Mood and Affect

Mood is defined as the underlying, more stable emotional tone, and affect is the quick reactivity of emotions depending on external circumstances or topics of interest. If we observe and listen well during the discussion of the chief complaint, the patient will likely have provided us already with a good understanding of the underlying mood.

We notice the range (how many different emotions are on display) and the intensity (depth of each single emotion, from barely any facial display of emotion to highly intense, hysterical or dramatic). Is the emotion displayed appropriate for the subject of discussion or is the affect incongruent (eg, the person is laughing while relaying a sad or traumatic event)?

Hallucinations

Auditory hallucinations are the most common type of hallucination in psychiatric disorders.

In the case of visual, tactile, gustatory, or somatic hallucinations, clinicians must consider the possibility of an underlying physical disease, such as the delirium, and a medical workup should be pursued immediately. Dissociation and post-traumatic stress disorder (PTSD) can cause a variety of perceptual disturbances, including all forms of hallucinations and flashbacks.

Delusions

Delusions are systems of perception that do not conform with our ordinary sense of reality. A common example is paranoia. In the United States, a common paranoid delusion would be of being followed or monitored by the Federal Bureau of Investigation (FBI) or Central Intelligence Agency (CIA), or families or hospital staff wishing the patient harm. The content of the delusion can provide clues toward diagnosis. A patient who is grandiose and says he is superman is likely manic. Someone who feels guilty for ruining their whole family is most likely depressed. Delusions take many forms and are influenced by culture. They can be somatic in nature (eg, inhabited by aliens or having microchips implanted), olfactory and gustatory. In Capgras delusions, the patient is convinced that their family has been replaced by imposters.

Suicidal Ideation and Non-Suicidal Self-Injurious Behaviors

Assessing every patient for SI is one of the most crucial parts of any psychiatric interview. Over the last 2 decades and especially since the COVID 19 pandemic, we have seen a steep increase in suicide attempts as well as completed suicides.[8] Many people present to emergency departments with new-onset or chronic SI.

For many patients, this is a very intimate, at times embarrassing experience (when the SI is ego-dystonic). However, SI can be very ego-syntonic and is often tied to hopelessness and the sense of a foreshortened future.

It is important for clinicians to feel comfortable asking about SI. The best approach is usually to leave questions about SI and urges to self-injure with intent to harm but not kill the body to a later point in the interview, when a relationship with the patient has been established, and the patient feels more comfortable. We need to ask. If the presence of SI has been affirmed, we must go into more details. Are these new ideas? Or chronic? Have they gotten worse recently? Is a particular stressor causing the worsening/origination of SIs? Is it passive ideation, such as wishing to not wake up? Is it active ideation with a plan? With what method? What is stopping them? Is there a history of past attempts? Do they feel hopeless? Are there protective factors (such as family, spirituality/religion, children, pets, and purpose in life)? Do they have strong, irresistible urges to go through with attempting suicide?

It is also important to ask if our patient feels safe right now while in the hospital ED.[9]

Much thought has gone into predicting people most at risk for suicide attempt, but criteria remain somewhat elusive.[10] Any patient who endorses SI or non-suicidal self-injurious urges will benefit from creation of a safety plan and referral to a mental health specialist, if discharged from the ED (**Table 1**: Suicide assessment).

Violence assessment

Aggression and agitation are frequent occurrences in several acute medical and psychiatric disorders. Therefore, the risk for violence is an integral part of the initial psychiatric interview.

Every patient should be assessed for current violent ideation and intention, especially homicidal intent. Past histories of arrest for violent crimes, history of frequent fights, and access to guns and other weapons need to be obtained. Single male patients with histories of violence, past arrests, substance use disorders, and multiple suicide attempts are at higher risk for violent behavior.[11] The management of agitation in the ED includes verbal de-escalation, pharmacological interventions, and restraints.

The cognitive examination

Assessing cognitive function is another crucial piece of a thorough clinical interview in both medical and psychiatric disorders.

Educational achievements or jobs held can provide us with information on the general level of intelligence and baseline functioning of the patient.

Orientation and level of alertness can give us hints of neurologic abnormalities such as minor strokes and mild cognitive impairment, dementia, or delirium.

Careful listening to the way patients tell their story and present their symptoms gives us insight into their ability to generalize, abstract, think logically, and use executive functioning. Being able to recall phone numbers, insurance information, addresses and other biographical details, or recent news items gives insight into short- and long-term memory.

Table 1
Suicide Assessment Five-Step Evaluation and Triage suicide risk assessment

Risk Factors	Suicidality
• History of suicide attempts or self-injurious: ideation behavior • Current mood disorder, psychotic disorder, ADHD, TBI, PTSD, cluster B personality disorder, conduct disorder • Current anhedonia, impulsivity, hopelessness panic, global insomnia, command auditory hallucinations • Family history of completed suicide, suicide attempts, or active episode requiring hospitalization • Recent stressors leading to shame or despair medical illness, intoxication, family turmoil, history of abuse, social isolation • Access to fire arms	• Ideation • Intent • Means (more or less lethal?) • Plan • Behaviors, including preparatory acts, self-injury, or suicide attempt

Protective Factors	Formulation of Risk
• No current suicidal ideation self-injurious behavior • Coping skills, religious beliefs, frustration tolerance • Responsibility to others, positive therapeutic relationships, social support • Thinking, planning about/for the future • Significant evidence of malingering or secondary gain	• Low • Medium • High Treatment Plan: • Minimal risk, no further action required • Hold for further observation • Refer to new/existing outpatient provider • Develop a safety plan • Acute inpatient psychiatric admission

The Montreal Cognitive Assessment[12] and Mini Mental Status Examination[13] assess basic attention, concentration, working memory, immediate recall, short-term memory, visuospatial abilities, orientation to person, time and place, and language functions. Both tests can be administered in about 10 minutes. However, they are coarse instruments and will only alert to major cognitive impairment. Some items on these cognitive screening tests are sensitive to cultural background, education level, and language competence in English.

Insight and Judgment

Any psychiatric assessment in the ED must include the dimensions of insight and judgment.

Insight is generally defined narrowly as whether the patient understands the nature of his condition. A psychotic patient, who has paranoid delusions of the FBI/CIA or similar government organization following him/her, may lack any insight and determine his actions from his delusional belief.

Out of insight flows judgment or the ability to manage one's health conditions and function in one's life and the world. Will the patient fill the prescription we are giving them? Are they able to organize themselves enough to follow through on outpatient recommendations or return to family and work?

Insight and judgment improve or impair prognosis. They can be disrupted by many different factors, such as the acute psychiatric condition, lack of education/medical understanding, cultural differences (eg, belief in alternative causes for illness such as spirits), cognitive deficits, and personality disorders.

Several scales have been developed to aid physicians in assessing psychiatric illness and can be accessed free of charge (**Table 2**: Freely accessed scales).

PHASE 3: ASSESSMENT AND PLAN: SUMMARY

In the final third phase of the interview, the diagnostic impression and next steps toward treatment (outpatient/inpatient) have in most cases become clear from the preceding interview. The suspected diagnosis should be shared with the patient in most situations. Depending on the nature of the problem, this may require a kind approach. The patient should be given time and space to ask questions, and findings should be explained in everyday language rather than medical terminology. This is also often a good time for psychoeducation on the existing issue or disorder. Many mental health issues are still surrounded by stigma, and many people do not know what is happening to them.[14]

The Trauma-Informed Interview

Every interview should be a trauma-informed interview. Many patients, who present to the ED, have significant histories of emotional, physical, or sexual trauma. This includes acute physical traumas, such as accidents as well as chronic, interpersonal traumas, including childhood abuse or a history of rape or molestation. Past histories of trauma increase health and mental health burden.[15] Therefore, the principles of trauma-informed care should be practiced in every interview. These principles are based on patient empowerment, choice, collaboration and safety, trustworthiness, and transparency. Sensitivity and respect and a patient-centered attitude should always be practiced.

Acute traumas such as a car accident or grave medical diagnoses will cause acute anxiety and stress reactions in many people in the immediate aftermath of the traumatic event. It is advisable to allow the patient to process their experience freely, or not at all,[16] depending on their preference.

Table 2
Helpful Screening Scales and Tools

General Screening	WHO-5, PHQ9, CGI	Five or Nine Questions, Respectively
Suicide assessment	CSSRS, Safe-T	5 questions, Safe-T expands with 6 items
	Safety Plan	Planning safe behaviors for a patient with SI to be discharged
Mania	YMRS (Young Mania Rating Scale)	11 items
Depression	Beck Depression Inventory, CES-D	21 or 20 self-report items, respectively
Anxiety	HAM-A	7 items or 14, respectively
Cognitive functions dementia	MMSE, MoCA	30 points, clinician administered
Psychosis	PSYRATS	Not frequently used in ED settings
Alcohol withdrawal	CIWA	10 items, aides in management of withdrawal
Opiate withdrawal	COWS	11 items, scores severity of opiate withdrawal
Catatonia	Bush-Francis Catatonia Rating Scale	Clinician administered, 23 items

CSSRS: The Columbia-Suicide Severity Rating Scale: Initial Validity and Internal Consistency Findings From Three Multisite Studies with Adolescents and Adults. K Posner PhD, GK Brown PhD et al. Am J Psychiatry. 2011 Dec: 168(12): 1266-1277.

Safe-T: Suicide Assessment Five-Step Evaluation and Triage SAFE-T Pocket Card. Suicide Prevention Resource Center. 2009.

Safety Plan: Stanley-Brown Safety Planning Intervention. www.suicidesafetyplan.com.

YMRS: Young RC, Biggs JT, Ziegler VE, Meyer DA. A rating scale for mania: reliability, validity and sensitivity. Br J Psychiatry. 1978;133:429-435.

Beck Depression Inventory: Beck AT, Ward CH, Mendelson M, Erbaugh J. (1961) An inventory for measuring depression. Arch Gen Psych, 4, 561-571.

Commonly Used Scales

CES-D: Radloff LS. (1977). The CES-D scale: A self-report depression scale for research in the general population. Applied Psychological Measurements, 1, 385-401.

HAM-A: Hamilton M. The assessment of anxiety states by rating. Br J Med Psychol (1959);32:50-55. PSYRATS: The Psychotic Symptom Rating Scales: Their usefulness and properties in first episode psychosis. Drake R, Haddock G, et al. Schizophr Res. 2007 Jan;89(1–3):119-122.

CIWA: Sullivan JT, Sykora K, et al. Assessment of Alcohol withdrawal: The revised Clinical Institute Withdrawal Assessment for Alcohol scale (CIWA-Ar). Br J of Addiction 84:1353-1357, 1989.

COWS: The Clinical Opiate Withdrawal Scale. Wesson DR, Ling W. J Psychoactive Drugs. 2003 Apr-Jun;35(2):253-9.

Bush-Frances Catatonia Rating Scale: Rating scale and standardized examination. Acta Psychiatry Scand. 1996;93(2):129-136.

Abbreviations: CGI, Clinical Gobal Impressions Scale; MMSE, Mini Mental Status Exam; MoCA, Montreal Cognitive Assessment; PHQ9, Patient Health Questionnaire; TBI, Traumatic Brain Injury; WHO-5, Well Being Index-5.

Interpersonal or chronic traumas have powerful impact on formation of personality and relationship style. Frequently, people with trauma histories have had negative experiences with the medical system and place limited trust in medical providers. A respectful stance is again of particularly great benefit.

Chronic traumas should not be discussed in any first interview. This discussion should be reserved for a patient and their loved ones or therapist. If a patient spontaneously brings up traumatic history and memory, an empathic response towards the patient's suffering is warranted.

Post-traumatic stress disorder can present in a multitude of ways. It can present with high levels of panic and anxiety or emotional numbness. Patients can seem delirious or psychotic, when they are acutely dissociated. At other times, physiological activation is so high that they cannot sleep and seem manic. Depression is often co-morbid with chronic trauma.[15]

Women and men assaulted by intimate partners frequent the EDs at a higher rate.[17] If current domestic violence is suspected or confirmed, investigation should be followed with additional questions: Has the physical violence increased in the last 6 months? Has the abuser ever used or threatened you with a weapon? Do you believe (s)he is capable of killing you? Has (s)he beaten you while you were pregnant? Is (s)he violently and constantly jealous of you? A referral to a mental health team or police is often recommended and should be pursued with the patient's consent.

Challenging Interviews

Agitated, intoxicated, or nonverbal patients and persons with certain personality disorders may present additional challenges. Many patients are being brought to the ED by law enforcement or ambulance, often called by a family member or bystander. Some arrive in the ED, behaving aggressively or were agitated in public and have already been medicated in the ambulance for violent behavior. With agitated and combative patients, the first and most immediate concern must be the safety of all staff and patients.

Intoxication is one of the frequent causes for emergency department visits and agitation. At times, patients are too intoxicated even to participate in an interview. Investigation about the use of addictive medications and substance use is vital for any psychiatric (and medical) interview. Type of substance(s) used, frequency of use, last use before visit, history of withdrawal symptoms, and complications (such as delirium tremens, seizures, other medical complications) need to be investigated. Neglecting to pursue this line of questions may lead to medical emergencies such as seizures or delirium.

If patients have taken an overdose in suicidal intent, it is particularly important to investigate the details of the attempt, substance taken, as quickly as possible to avoid further worsening/death.

Patients with opiate dependence may repeatedly present to the ED with complaints of severe pain, seeking renewal of opiate prescriptions.

In the presence of an agitated patient, the main interview may be the observation of behavior and spontaneous verbalization. What is the patient yelling? Does he sound paranoid? Is speech slurred and dysarthric? Is he twitching and tweaking (often signs of intoxication with amphetamines or large amounts of cocaine/crack)? Does he seem "frozen," as seen in patients with catatonia or severe opiate intoxication?

Patients who are nonverbal present an obvious challenge to the examining doctor. We rely heavily on verbal information in making a diagnosis and forming a treatment plan, although careful physical examination and observation of the behavior of a nonverbal patient still provide us with important information. Does he seem under severe tension, intermittently moving in repetitive patterns, or demonstrate increased rigidity such as in catatonia? The Bush Francis Catatonia Rating scale[18] is a helpful tool in diagnosing this emergency medical condition. This should be followed by a medical workup to exclude neuroleptic malignant syndrome and other medical causes.

Another cause for remaining mute is an acutely dissociated state as might be triggered by traumatic events. Family may report normal functioning up to a triggering event and then abrupt onset of symptoms.

If no outside information is available, careful observation over time can often help with establishing the correct diagnosis. Medical evaluation should proceed as quickly as possible with blood tests, physical examination EKG, urine tests, and especially toxicology screen.

Personality disorders can be challenging to diagnose in an initial emergency room interview but may influence the patient's relationship to the treatment team and adherence to proposed interventions. Patients with personality disorders may elicit powerful feelings (counter transference) in providers because of their challenging relationship style. Diagnosis of a personality disorder in the ED is unnecessary, however.

The most challenging personality disorders are those of cluster B: borderline, antisocial, and narcissistic personality disorder.

A common reason for patients with borderline personality disorder to present to the ED is an increase in self-injurious urges/behavior or worsening SI.

Patients with antisocial personality disorder may have ulterior motives for their presentation, different from the stated chief complaint.

In patients with narcissistic personality disorder, their feelings of entitlement and their devaluing or idealizing may elicit counter transference in the treating provider. If possible, management of such patients should be referred to trained mental health providers.

SUMMARY

In psychiatry, the patient interview is generally still the most important tool for establishing a diagnosis. Since the advent of the DSM and ICD diagnostic systems of descriptive diagnoses, the structure of a typical psychiatric interview, especially in the emergency department setting, has changed significantly from prior, more psychodynamic interview formats. Eliciting symptoms will provide the set of data necessary to make a descriptive diagnosis. Unfortunately, some of the finer points of bio-psychosocial formulations will often not be caught by adhering to the format outlined above. They are still part of the art of interviewing, which can be improved and mastered with practice and genuine interest in the human being before us.

CLINICS CARE POINTS

- A thorough clinical interview helps establish diagnosis, psychiatric, or otherwise.
- Parts of the interview are observations of nonverbal clues, behavior, and appearance.
- A noncooperative patient will still provide much valuable information when observed.
- The interview is a crucial tool in building a collaborative treatment relationship with a patient.
- The experience of empathic listening improves outcomes and adherence to recommended treatments and reduces burnout in clinicians.
- Good histories lead to precise diagnosis and improve outcomes.

REFERENCES

1. Trzeciak S, Mazzarelli A. Compassionomics, the revolutionary scientific evidence that caring makes a difference. Pensacola, FL: Studer Group Publishing LLC; 2019.
2. Beckman HB, Frankel RM. The effect of physician behavior on the collection of data. Ann Intern Med 1984;101(5):692–6.
3. Detsky AS. Learning the art and science of diagnosis. JAMA 2022;237(18): 1759–60.
4. MacKinnon RA, Michels R, Buckley PJ. The psychiatric interview in clinical practice. Third edition. Washington, DC: American Psychiatric Association Publishing; 2016.
5. Carlat DJ. The psychiatric interview: a practical guide. Second Edition. Philadelphia, PA: Lippincott Williams&Wilkins; 2005.
6. Sullivan HS. The psychiatric interview, a guide for therapists and other interviewers, by the founder of the interpersonal psychiatry. New York, NY: WW Norton & Company; 1970.
7. The psychiatric interview in the emergency department. Emergency Clinics of North America 2000;18(2):173–83.
8. Suicide worldwide in 2019, global health estimates. Geneva, Switzerland: World Health Organization; 2021.
9. Feinstein R, Plutchik R. Violence and suicide assessment scale in the psychiatric emergency room. Compr Psychiatr 1990;3(4):337–43.
10. Belsher BE, Smolenski DJ, Pruitt LD, et al. Prediction models for suicide attempts and deaths: a systematic review and simulation. JAMA Psychiatr 2019;76(6): 642–51.
11. Lawrence RE, Fuchs B, Krumheuer A, et al. Self-harm during visits to the emergency department: a qualitative content analysis. J Acad Consultation-Liaison Psychiatry 2022;63:3.
12. Nasreddine ZS, Phillips NA, Bédirian V, et al. The Montreal Cognitive Assessment, MoCA: a brief screening tool for mild cognitive impairment. J Am Geriatr Soc 2005;53(4):695–9.
13. The mini-mental Status Examinnation: a comprehensive review. J Am Geriatr Soc 1992;40(9):922–35.
14. Corrigan PW, Morris SB, Michaels PJ, et al. Challenging the public stigma of mental illness: a meta-analysis of outcome studies. Psychiatr Serv 2012;63(10): 963–73.
15. Heim C, Jeffrey Newport D, Mletzko T, et al. The link between childhood trauma and depression: insights from HPA axis studies in humans. Psychoneuroendocrinology Elsevier 2008;33(6):693–710.
16. Center for Preparedness and Response, Center for Disease Control and Prevention: 6 Guiding Principles to a Trauma-Informed Approach. Available at: https://www.cdc.gov/cpr/infographics/6-principles_trauma_info.htm. Accessed 2015.
17. Snyder C, Webster D, O'Sullivan CS, et al. Intimate partner violence: development of a brief assessment for the emergency department. Acad Emerg Med 2009;16(11):1208–16.
18. Bush G, Fink M, Petrides G, et al. Catatonia. I. Rating scale and standardized examination. Acta Psychiatr Scand 1996;93(2):129–36.

Management of the Agitated Patient

Carmen Wolfe, MD[a],*, Nicole McCoin, MD[b]

KEYWORDS

- Agitation • Physical restraints • Antipsychotics • Benzodiazepines • Sedation

KEY POINTS

- Non-coercive de-escalation strategies should be utilized primarily in all patient populations.
- Physical restraints should be utilized with caution given their safety risks, with close attention to patient safety and required documentation.
- Clinicians must select an optimal pharmacologic strategy based on each individual patient presentation given the heterogeneity of evidence for medications utilized for chemical restraint.

INTRODUCTION

Management of acutely agitated and combative patients is a key component of care in the emergency department (ED). While rates vary among facilities, one urban ED noted the prevalence of agitation to be 2.6% of all patients, with 84% requiring physical restraint and 72% requiring chemical restraint.[1] Determining the etiology of the patient's agitation is of utmost importance given the broad differential including underlying neurologic, infectious, toxicologic, metabolic, and psychiatric disorders. In order to facilitate this evaluation, physicians must control the patient's symptoms with options including non-pharmacologic and pharmacologic interventions.

NON-PHARMACOLOGIC INTERVENTIONS
Noncoercive Deescalation

While the management of agitation traditionally focuses on the use of physical and chemical restraints, the utilization of a non-coercive approach should be a primary focus.[2] The American Association for Emergency Psychiatry created Project BETA (Best practices in the Evaluation and Treatment of Agitation), which provides helpful

---

[a] Department of Emergency Medicine, Tristar Skyline Medical Center, 3443 Dickerson Pike, Suite 230, Nashville, TN 37207, USA; [b] Department of Emergency Medicine, Ochsner Medical Center, 1514 Jefferson Highway, New Orleans, LA 70121, USA
* Corresponding author.
E-mail address: carmen.wolfe@hcahealthcare.com

Emerg Med Clin N Am 42 (2024) 13–29
https://doi.org/10.1016/j.emc.2023.06.010
0733-8627/24/© 2023 Elsevier Inc. All rights reserved.

guidance in this arena.[3] These guidelines focus on a three-step method. First, the patient is verbally engaged. Second, a collaborative relationship is established. Finally, the patient is verbally de-escalated. To accomplish these goals, ten domains are proposed and explored, with keys for implementation for each. See **Table 1** for a brief summary of the BETA recommendations.[3]

Show of Force

Some agitated patients may respond well to a show of force by security personnel. Permanent security installations such as metal detectors, wands, and security cameras have been shown to be perceived as increasing safety by patients with ED, and may help to deter violence in agitated patients.[4]

Physical Restraints

When attempts at other non-pharmacologic interventions have failed, the physician may need to temporarily utilize physical restraints. A small cross-sectional study found that restraints are utilized in 0.5% of ED visits.[5] A predominant number were male (66.7%) and had a history of psychiatric illness (61.9%), with a cluster analysis revealing 2 specific cohorts: a younger male population presenting with substance use-related chief complaints and an older population presenting with medical concerns.[5] More than demographic characteristics, presenting symptoms are more likely to predict the need for physical restraints and including arrival in restraints, arrival in the evening or at night, or presentations with mania, disruptive behavior, psychosis, or impaired insight.[6]

A wide variety of physical restraints may be utilized including limb restraints and restraining belts or vests. Other forms of physical restraints may be utilized in less mobile patients such as extreme incline of the bed, locked bed rails, or sheets tucked tightly around the patient, though these methods are more commonly utilized in non-emergent settings within nursing facilities.[7]

When the decision is made to utilize physical restraints in the emergent setting, a standardized approach should be employed. A sufficient team would ideally consist of at least 5 individuals: one leader and one person to restrain each limb by placing pressure above the knees and around the elbow. Restraints should be placed on all 4 limbs initially, as restraining only 1 or 2 limbs may result in a twisting injury or increase the risk of flipping a bed. Leg restraints should be secured to the opposite corner of the bed frame, and never to bed rails which have the potential to move. Arm restraints should be secured to the ipsilateral side of the bedframe with one arm above the head and one arm secured to the side. This pattern of restraint limits the patient's ability to generate momentum when rocking the bed and decreases the risk of a flipping injury.

Patient positioning during restraint is also paramount to consider for patient safety. The "hobble" or "hog-tie" has been shown in study populations to restrict pulmonary function.[8] Pillows should be removed, and the prone position should be avoided. When patients are in the supine position, the head of the bed should be elevated to reduce the risk of aspiration. Finally, careful attention to patient position should be utilized to minimize risk of pressure-related injuries.

Physical restraints should be discontinued as soon as it is safe to do so. Depending on the patient's level of cooperation, it may be wise to remove the restraints in a stepwise fashion. When moving from four-point to two-point restraints, remove a contralateral arm and leg.

Table 1
Noncoercive de-escalation (holloman)

BETA 3 Step Method	Non-coercive De-escalation	
	Domains to Promote Success	Keys to Implementation
Step 1: Verbally Engage the Patient	Respect personal space	• Maintain two arms-length distance
	Do not be provocative	• Avoid unintended escalation
	Establish verbal contact	• A single person should interact with the patient
		• Begin with an introduction, then orientation and reassurance
Step 2: Establish a Collaborative Relationship	Be concise	• Keep it simple
		• Repetition is essential
	Establish wants and feelings	• Consider a broad range of physical and emotional wants
		• Utilize clues from the patient's comments and behaviors
	Listen closely to what the patient is saying	• Use active listening
		• Try to truly understand the perspective of the patient
	Agree or agree to disagree	• Attempt to agree: with the truth, in principle, or with the odds
		• If all else fails, agree to disagree
Step 3: Verbally De-escalate the Patient	Lay down the law and set clear limits	• Set limits in a respectful manner
		• Coach the patient in how to stay in control
	Offers choices and optimism	• Offer choices, including creature comforts
		• Broach the subject of medication
		• Provide hope
	Debrief the patient and staff	• Help the patient reflect on the sequence of events
		• Debrief with staff for future process improvement

PHARMACOLOGIC INTERVENTIONS
Route of Administration

Chemical restraint may be necessary in patients who do not respond to noncoercive deescalation techniques and is administered via either oral (PO), intramuscular (IM), or intravenous (IV) routes in most cases. Many factors determine the route of administration of medication. Oral administration of medications is feasible in patients who are cooperative enough to comply with treatment. Studies that demonstrate the effectiveness of oral medication in the management of acute agitation either required consent for oral treatment from the patient or, at minimum, that the patient was willing to take the oral medication. Thus these studies do not represent the full scope of agitation that may be seen, particularly those who are severely agitated and require swift and efficient chemical restraint in order to assure that the patient and staff are not harmed.[9] The choice of IM versus IV administration should be made based on the clinician's best judgment regarding which will be the safest route of administration for both the patient and the staff.

PHARMACOLOGIC OPTIONS
Typical Antipsychotics

Haloperidol (Haldol) and droperidol (Inapsine) are typical (first generation) antipsychotics in the butyrophenone class and primarily exert their effect as a dopamine (D2) receptor antagonist. These medications have minimal effects on a patient's hemodynamic status; minimal anticholinergic activity; and minimal medication interactions. However, they do have notable side effects. QTc prolongation can occur with the administration of both haloperidol and droperidol. In fact, in 2001, the FDA issued a black box warning regarding the use of droperidol and the risk of QTc prolongation and Torsades de Pointes. There has been much controversy over this which culminated in a position statement by the American Academy of Emergency Medicine in 2015 that asserted that, although the black box warning is still in place by the FDA, intramuscular doses of up to 10 mg of droperidol seem to be as safe and effective as other medications used for the sedation of agitated patients.[10] A Cochrane review in 2016 further supported this finding, with high quality evidence to support its use.[11] In comparison to haloperidol, droperidol leads to faster control of the patient, more consistent sedation, a shorter duration of effect (half-life of haloperidol 18 hours vs half-life of droperidol of 2.3 hours), and less extrapyramidal side effects.[12] Haloperidol and droperidol can cause extrapyramidal side effects including dystonia, which can be treated with diphenhydramine or benztropine. Haloperidol and droperidol can also lower seizure threshold and cause neuroleptic malignant syndrome. They should be avoided in Parkinson's disease, in patients presenting with anticholinergic toxidromes, and utilized with caution in pregnancy and lactating females.[13]

Atypical Antipsychotics

Atypical (second generation) antipsychotics are dopamine (D2) receptor antagonists and serotonin-2A (5-HT2A) receptor antagonists (among other receptors). This difference in mechanism of action leads to fewer extrapyramidal side effects than typical antipsychotics. These agents tend to provide more tranquilization than sedation compared with typical antipsychotics.

Ziprasidone (Geodon) was the first atypical antipsychotic medication to become available in an IM formulation.[14] Utilization of ziprasidone is associated with a lower likelihood of extrapyramidal symptoms, postural hypotension, and anticholinergic symptoms.[15] It is associated with a mild, transient hyperprolactinemia.[15] Studies focused on the ED utilization of this medication are limited with mixed results when compared to other antipsychotic and benzodiazepines.[16–18]

Olanzapine (Zyprexa) is FDA approved in IM and oral-dissolving formulations for the management of agitation associated with bipolar I mania and schizophrenia. In comparison with the typical antipsychotics, there is less concern for extrapyramidal side effects, neuroleptic malignant syndrome, and QTc prolonging effects with olanzapine administration. However, patients may demonstrate anticholinergic effects, orthostatic hypotension, and synergistic effects with other CNS depressants. There is also an FDA Box Warning regarding the use of olanzapine and increased mortality in elderly patients with dementia-related psychosis. Therefore, olanzapine use may be most appropriate in the younger patient with agitation that appears to be primarily driven by underlying psychiatric disease, as opposed to the undifferentiated agitated or combative patient whose presentation may be more greatly attributed to other medical comorbidities or intoxication.

Intravenous use of olanzapine is off-label. However, its use has been explored for the management of acute agitation, particularly during national shortages of typical antipsychotics. The most significant concern with IV olanzapine was whether rates of respiratory depression were higher with its use compared to either the IM formulation of olanzapine or typical antipsychotics. A meta-analysis revealed that rates of respiratory depression and airway obstruction were low and similar to that of these other agents, including IM olanzapine, however its use is controversial, and further studies are warranted to fully explore its safety.[19]

Risperidone (Risperdal) is administered in an oral disintegrating, oral solution, or IM depot form. Similar to olanzapine, there is an FDA Box Warning precluding its use in dementia-related psychosis. Also, like olanzapine, it is used in patients with agitation that is likely due to underlying psychiatric disease, particularly schizophrenia. In particular, risperidone may be an option when the patient can comply with an oral medication option given its onset of action is more rapid than other medications with oral formulations.[20] Time to peak plasma concentration of risperidone is 1.5 hours compared to 6 hours with oral olanzapine.[21]

Benzodiazepines

Benzodiazepines exert their effects at the GABA receptor leading to sedation, anxiolysis, and anterograde amnesia. This class of medication is often used when the etiology of agitation is unknown or when agitation is due to drug intoxication or withdrawal. Benzodiazepines can also be effective in acute psychosis. While patients experience less extrapyramidal side effects with the use of benzodiazepines in comparison with antipsychotics, benzodiazepine administration may cause excessive sedation, respiratory depression and hypotension, particularly in the presence of other sedating medications. There is an FDA Box Warning regarding the concomitant use of benzodiazepines and opioids due to risk of over-sedation, respiratory depression, and even death. Paradoxic disinhibition with findings of increased talkativeness, excitement, and emotions as well as excessive movements may be seen in less than 1% of patients.[22]

Clinicians may use lorazepam (Ativan) or midazolam (Versed) as options for the treatment of the acutely agitated patient. Compared with lorazepam, midazolam provides the benefit of more rapid onset of sedation followed by a shorter time to arousal.[23] Thus, the clinician must weigh the options of either administering midazolam with the anticipation of a shorter onset of action/shorter duration of action or administering lorazepam with the anticipation of a longer onset of action/longer duration of action. Although midazolam may lead to a more rapid onset of sedation, its use may be more likely to require additional medications to maintain sedation.[17,18] Combination with an antipsychotic medication should therefore be considered if midazolam is chosen and prolonged sedation is desired.[24] Given the increasing length and frequency of benzodiazepine shortages over the recent years, it is prudent for the emergency physician to be familiar with characteristics of multiple formulations and routes of administration.[25]

Ketamine

Ketamine is a dissociative anesthetic and exerts multiple effects including affecting opioid receptors, nitric oxide synthetase, and as an NMDA receptor antagonist. It may be used as a first line agent for agitation, or may be administered if other treatments have not yet achieved desired sedation.[26–28] Although recent studies demonstrate that ketamine appears to rapidly control agitation while maintaining similar rates of adverse events compared to other agents, it is effectively procedural sedation and thus requires the corresponding appropriate level of monitoring. If given following the failure of other agents to achieve desired sedation, it may be prudent to reduce the ketamine dose by 50%. Ketamine has a short time to the onset and short duration of action as well, which may lead to need for redosing or administration of additional medications. Side effects include hypertension, tachycardia, hypersalivation, laryngospasm, apnea, vomiting, and dysphoric emergence phenomena.[29] In patients with a known history of schizophrenia, ketamine should be used with caution due to the risk of exacerbation of psychosis symptoms including hallucinations and delusions (**Table 2**).[30]

Given the many options available, the clinician could choose from a variety of agents depending on the particular patient presentation (**Table 2**). These options, in general, include first generation antipsychotic alone, second generation antipsychotic alone, benzodiazepine alone, a combination of first or second generation antipsychotic and a benzodiazepine, or ketamine (typically given when one or more of the above have failed to achieve adequate sedation). Multiple studies have examined these combination treatment approaches, and are summarized in **Table 3**. Assessing the available evidence points to several trends. The combination of an antipsychotic and benzodiazepine consistently outperforms use of single agents, with the exception of ketamine. When selecting an antipsychotic, droperidol often outperforms other drugs in single agent trials and is often the drug of choice given its more rapid onset. When selecting a benzodiazepine, midazolam consistently performs well in trials and also offers a faster onset of action. The multitude of outcome measures, medications, dosage, and routes of administration make it difficult to draw a single conclusion from analysis of these studies, and point to the need for further targeted research in the emergency setting.[32]

Utilization of adjunct medications

Diphenhydramine is commonly added to a combination of haloperidol 5 mg and lorazepam 2 mg for the treatment of acute agitation in a formation known colloquially as a "B52." A retrospective review does not support the addition of diphenhydramine, showing no difference in need for additional sedation. The diphenhydramine group also had more oxygen desaturation, hypotension, use of physical restraints, and a longer length of stay. Patients who did not receive the diphenhydramine had a higher likelihood of receiving an antimuscarinic within the following 48 hours, though none had documented extrapyramidal symptoms.[40]

UNIQUE CONSIDERATIONS FOR SPECIAL POPULATIONS
Pediatrics

Psychiatric concerns have been estimated to account for 2% to 5% of pediatric ED visits, with incidence increasing year after year.[41–43] As with adults, nonpharmacologic interventions should be emphasized in pediatric populations. In the event that chemical sedation is necessary, it is prudent to note that pediatric patients may have a paradoxic reaction to diphenhydramine or benzodiazepines, leading to increased agitation.[22,44] If physical restraints are required, time requirements for initiation and renewal of restraints are more stringent for pediatrics. The Joint Commission

Table 2
Pharmacologic interventions: medication characteristics[31]

Class	Generic Name	Available Routes of Administration	Typical Initial Dose Range	Onset of Action	Duration of Action	Special Considerations
Typical Antipsychotics	Haloperidol	PO, IM, IV	2-5 mg PO; 5-10 mg IM/IV	10 min IM/IV	4-6 h	Extrapyramidal side effects; QTc prolongation; lowers seizure threshold; can cause neuroleptic malignant syndrome
	Droperidol	IM, IV	1.25-2.5 mg IM/IV	3-5 min IM/IV	2-4 h	
Atypical Antipsychotics	Olanzapine	PO (disintegrating tablet), IM	2.5-10 mg PO, 5-10 mg IM	15-120 min PO, 10-30 min IM	6-8 h	Better for young patients with pure psychiatric presentations; synergistic with other CNS depressants; black box warning in dementia-related psychosis
	Risperidone	PO (disintegrating tablet, oral solution)	1-3 mg PO	30-120 min PO	4-6 h	Primarily used in schizophrenia; short time to peak effect
	Ziprasidone	PO, IM	20-40 mg PO, 10-20 mg IM	15-30 min IM	6-8 h	Lower risk of extrapyramidal symptoms
Benzodiazepines	Lorazepam	PO, IM, IV	0.5-2 mg PO, 1-2 mg IM	15-30 min PO/IM	2-6 h	Used in undifferentiated agitation or agitation due to drug intoxication/withdrawal; longer time to onset of action/longer duration in comparison to midazolam
	Midazolam	IM, IV	2-5 mg IM	2-10 min IM	30-90 min	Used in undifferentiated agitation or agitation due to drug intoxication/withdrawal; relatively short onset time; relatively rapid time to arousal
Other	Ketamine	IM, IV	4-5 mg/kg IM, 1-2 mg/kg IV	2-4 min IM, 1-2 min IV	5-30 min	Side effects include hypertension, tachycardia, hypersalivation, laryngospasm, vomiting, and emergence reaction; could cause agitation in patients with schizophrenia; consider dose reduction if co-administered with other agents

Pharmacologic Interventions for Acute Agitation in Adults: Medication Characteristics

Table 3
A comparison of pharmacologic options for acute agitation

		Pharmacologic Interventions: Evidence for Utilization			
Study Type	Trial Description	Authors	Comparison Groups	Outcomes	Caveats
Comparison of Single Agent Antipsychotics					
Retrospective Observational	Rescue sedation when treating acute agitation in the emergency department with intramuscular antipsychotics	Klein et al.[18] 2019	Droperidol 5–10 mg vs Haloperidol 5–10 mg vs Olanzapine 10 mg	Need for rescue medication lower for olanzapine and droperidol compared with haloperidol	Retrospective study; possibly confounded by the co-administration of other medications
Prospective Randomized	Droperidol vs haloperidol for chemical restraint of agitated and combative patients	Thomas et al.[12] 1992	Haloperidol 5 mg IM/IV vs Droperidol 5 mg IM/IV	Decreased combativeness at 10 and 30 min with IM droperidol vs IM haloperidol; no significant difference when comparing IV route	Small study size (n = 68)
RCT	Droperidol v. haloperidol for the sedation of aggressive behavior in acute mental health	Calver et al.[34] 2015	Droperidol 10 mg IM vs Haloperidol 10 mg IM	No significant difference in median time to sedation, though additional sedation used more often with haloperidol (13% vs 5%)	Adverse effects less common with haloperidol (1% vs 5%)

Benzodiazepines vs Antipsychotics (Single Agents)

RCT	Management of acute undifferentiated agitation in the emergency department: a randomized double-blind trial of droperidol, ziprasidone, and midazolam	Martel et al.[17] 2005	Droperidol 5 mg IM vs Ziprasidone 20 mg IM vs Midazolam 5 mg IM	Midazolam cohort was more likely to require rescue medication to achieve adequate sedation	No difference in respiratory depression
RCT	Randomized double-blind trial of intramuscular droperidol, ziprasidone, and lorazepam for acute undifferentiated agitation in the emergency department	Martel et al.[16] 2021	Droperidol 5 mg IM vs Ziprasidone 10 mg IM vs Ziprasidone 20 mg IM vs Lorazepam 2 mg IM	Droperidol was more effective at achieving adequate sedation at 15 min than ziprasidone or lorazepam	Respiratory depression was lower with droperidol
Prospective Observational	Intramuscular midazolam, olanzapine, ziprasidone, or haloperidol for treating acute agitation in the emergency department	Klein et al.[33] 2018	Haloperidol 5 mg IM vs Haloperidol 10 mg IM vs Ziprasidone 20 mg IM vs Olanzapine 10 mg IM vs Midazolam 5 mg IM	Midazolam cohort with more effective sedation at 15 min than haloperidol, ziprasidone, and olanzapine	No difference in adverse events

(continued on next page)

Table 3
(continued)

		Pharmacologic Interventions: Evidence for Utilization			
Study Type	Trial Description	Authors	Comparison Groups	Outcomes	Caveats
RCT	A prospective, double-blind, randomized trial of midazolam vs haloperidol vs lorazepam in the chemical restraint of violent and severely agitated patients	Nobay et al.[23] 2014	Haloperidol 5 mg IM vs Lorazepam 2 mg IM vs Midazolam 5 mg IM	Midazolam with shorter time of sedation onset and shorter time to arousal than lorazepam or haloperidol	No difference in adverse events
Benzodiazepines vs Antipsychotics (combinations)					
RCT	Haloperidol, lorazepam, or both for psychotic agitation? A multicenter, prospective, double-blind, emergency department study	Battaglia, J et al.[35] 1997	Lorazepam 2 mg IM vs Haloperidol 5 mg IM vs Lorazepam 2 mg IM + Haloperidol 5 mg IM	Tranquilization most rapid with lorazepam/haloperidol combination rather than either agent alone; side effects did not differ significantly between treatment arms	Patients treated with haloperidol alone did have more extrapyramidal side effects
RCT	A double-blind study of lorazepam vs the combination of haloperidol and lorazepam in managing agitation	Bieniek, S et al.[36] 1998	Lorazepam 2 mg IM vs Lorazepam 2 mg IM + Haloperidol 5 mg IM	Combination of lorazepam and haloperidol had superior efficacy at controlling agitation, particularly notable at 60 min, compared to lorazepam alone	Small sample size; low power

RCT	Effect of Lorazepam With Haloperidol vs Haloperidol Alone on Agitated Delirium in Patients with Advanced Cancer Receiving Palliative Care: A Randomized Clinical Trial	Hui, D et al.[37] 2017	Lorazepam 3 mg IV + Haloperidol 2 mg IV vs Haloperidol 2 mg IV	Combination of lorazepam plus haloperidol led to greater decrease in agitation at 8 h compared to haloperidol alone	Study of hospitalized oncology patients (not either ED or Psychiatric ED environment); looked at endpoint at 8 h
RCT	Midazolam-Droperidol, Droperidol, or Olanzapine for Acute Agitation: A Randomized Clinical Trial	Taylor, D et al.[38] 2017	Midazolam 5 mg IV + Droperidol 5 mg IV vs Droperidol 5 mg IV vs Olanzapine 10 mg IV	Combination of midazolam and droperidol was superior to droperidol alone and olanzapine alone in achieving adequate sedation at 10 min and required fewer additional doses or alternative drugs to achieve adequate sedation	Adverse events between these three groups did not differ
RCT	Intravenous droperidol or olanzapine as an adjunct to midazolam for the acutely agitated patient: a multi-centered, randomized, double-blind, placebo-controlled clinical trial	Chan et al.[24] 2013	Midazolam 2.5–5 mg IV vs Droperidol 5 mg IV + Midazolam 2.5–5 mg IV vs Olanzapine 5 mg IV + Midazolam 2.5–5 mg IV	The addition of either droperidol or olanzapine to midazolam decreases time to adequate sedation, with no difference between those two groups	No difference in adverse event profiles or ED length of stay
Prospective Observational	Prospective study of haloperidol plus lorazepam vs	Thiemann et al.[39] 2022	Haloperidol 5 mg IM + Lorazepam 2 mg IM vs Droperidol 5 mg IM	Median time to sedation for droperidol plus midazolam was shorter	Patients in the droperidol plus midazolam group

(continued on next page)

Table 3
(continued)

Pharmacologic Interventions: Evidence for Utilization					
Study Type	**Trial Description**	**Authors**	**Comparison Groups**	**Outcomes**	**Caveats**
	droperidol plus midazolam for the treatment of acute agitation in the emergency department		IM + Midazolam 5 mg IM	(10 min) than haloperidol plus lorazepam (30 min)	were more likely to receive oxygen supplementation, but none required intubation
Ketamine vs Combination of Antipsychotic/Benzodiazepine					
RCT	Rapid Agitation Control With Ketamine in the Emergency Department: A Blinded, Randomized Controlled Trial	Barbic, D et al.[27] 2021	Ketamine 5 mg/kg IM vs Midazolam 5 mg IM + Haloperidol 5 mg IM	Shorter median time to sedation with ketamine (5.8 vs 14.7 min)	12.5% of patients experienced serious adverse events with ketamine vs 5% with midazolam/ haloperidol (not statistically significant difference; 80 patients enrolled [stopped early due to COVID-19])
RCT	Efficacy of ketamine for initial control of acute agitation in the emergency department: A randomized study	Lin et al.[28] 2021	Ketamine 4 mg/kg IM or 1 mg/kg IV vs Haloperidol 5–10 mg IM/IV + Lorazepam 1–2 mg IM/IV	Median time to sedation lower with ketamine (15 vs 36 min)	No significant adverse effects with ketamine

limits restraint orders to 1 hour for children under the age of 9, and 2 hours for children age 9 to 17.[45]

Pregnancy and Postpartum

Patients are at increased risk of an exacerbation of psychiatric illness during the perinatal period due to medication changes, withdrawal, and physiologic changes associated with pregnancy.[46] Physical restraint should be avoided if possible due to risk inferior vena cava compression in the supine position during the 2nd and 3rd trimesters.[47] Chemical sedation should be utilized with caution in this population due to potential teratogenicity as all antipsychotic medications cross the placenta.[48] A lack of controlled studies in pregnant women leaves clinicians with little high-quality data, and no antipsychotic has been definitively proven to be safe in pregnancy.[48] However, reports of congenital malformations associated with antipsychotics are very rare, and none have demonstrated causation.[48] Clinicians must weigh the risks of these medications, and the risk of patient harm from agitation often outweighs the risk of medication exposure in the emergent setting.[46] Risperidone and quetiapine are not known to be teratogenic and may be a prudent choice if the patent is willing to take an oral medication.[13,49] Expert consensus supports the use of haloperidol, second general antipsychotics, and benzodiazepines as needed for the management of acute agitation.[50]

Geriatrics

Elderly patients presenting to the emergency department with agitation or behavioral changes should be carefully evaluated given the wide spectrum of illness that may present with these symptoms. A standardized tool such as the Advanced Dementia Prognostic Tool (ADEPT) can guide clinicians through a careful evaluation.[51] By the Beers criteria, all antipsychotics are also potentially inappropriate, and the FDA has issued a black box warning for this class of medication in dementia-related psychosis due to increased mortality.[51] In the emergent setting, use of low dose olanzapine or risperidone carries the best consensus support.[51] Unless withdrawal is suspected, benzodiazepines should be avoided due to risk of prolonged sedation and paradoxic reaction in the elderly.[51] Diphenhydramine should be avoided due to its anticholinergic properties and risk of over-sedation.[52]

DOCUMENTATION AND LEGAL CONSIDERATIONS

The implementation of both pharmacologic and non-pharmacologic interventions has legal and ethical implications. The Department of Health and Human Services has published an extensive list of patient's rights detailing the conditions under which patient restraint is permissible.[45] The rationale for the implementation of restraints must include immediate danger to the patient or staff member, or others, and restraints must be discontinued at the earliest possible time.[45] Unless superseded by more restrictive State laws, the guidelines in this document govern documentation, timing for renewal, and training requirements related to restraints. When restraints are utilized, the patient must be evaluated face-to-face within 1 hour by a physician or other specifically trained provider. Restraint orders must be renewed every 4 hours, up to 24 hours, for adults. At the end of this time period, a new order for restraints must be placed.[45] Failure to follow these guidelines could results in adverse action for the physician or the hospital.

ETHICAL CONSIDERATIONS/PSYCHOLOGICAL COMPLICATIONS

It is important to consider the psychological impact of the use of restraints. Respect for patient autonomy must be prioritized, and patients should be included in the decision-making process as much as possible.[53] Patients report high rates of psychological distress after the utilization of common intervention such as physical restraints, being placed in seclusion, or being forced to take medication.[54] These experiences may impact future encounters with the healthcare system, either creating mistrust or acting as a deterrent for the patient who needs to seek care.

SUMMARY

Management of an agitated patient in the emergency department requires a team-based approach, keeping the patient's autonomy, safety, and medical well-being in the forefront of all considerations. Utilization of non-coercive de-escalation should be a priority, with the BETA recommendations offering a structured approach that can be followed by the staff team. If necessary, careful selection of an appropriate pharmacologic agent or combination should be selected by the physician for chemical restraint, with or without the addition of physical restraints as necessary for patient and staff safety. Careful documentation is necessary to ensure regulatory compliance.

CLINICS CARE POINTS

- Clinicians should follow a step-wise approach to the acutely agitated patient, beginning with non-coercive de-escalation strategies and moving on to pharmacologic interventions and physical restraints as necessary
- If chemical or physical restraint is utilized, clinicians must have a thorough understanding of the face-to-face examination, monitoring, and documentation requirements associated with the use of these restraints
- Given the heterogeneity in evidence regarding optimal medications for chemical restraints, clinicians should be familiar with multiple options and create a personalized plan for each patient as no single approach fits all presentations of agitation
- Common approaches include ketamine or a combination of a benzodiazepine and an antipsychotic, with the greatest evidence to support midazolam and droperidol
- Respect for the patient's autonomy, safety, and medical well-being must be at the forefront of the clinician's mind throughout the patient's management

DISCLOSURE

This research was supported (in whole or in part) by HCA Healthcare, United States and/or an HCA Healthcare affiliated entity. The views expressed in this publication represent those of the author(s) and do not necessarily represent the official views of HCA Healthcare or any of its affiliated entities.

REFERENCES

1. Miner JR, Klein LR, Cole JB, et al. The Characteristics and Prevalence of Agitation in an Urban County Emergency Department. Ann Emerg Med 2018;72(4): 361–70.
2. Richmond JS, Berlin JS, Fishkind AB, et al. Verbal de-escalation of the agitated patient: consensus statement of the American Association for Emergency

Psychiatry Project BETA De-escalation Workgroup. West J Emerg Med 2012; 13(1):17–25.

3. Holloman GH Jr, Zeller SL. Overview of Project BETA: Best practices in Evaluation and Treatment of Agitation. West J Emerg Med 2012;13(1):1–2.

4. McNamara R, Yu DK, Kelly JJ. Public perception of safety and metal detectors in an urban emergency department. Am J Emerg Med 1997;15(1):40–2.

5. Wong AH, Taylor RA, Ray JM, et al. Physical Restraint Use in Adult Patients Presenting to a General Emergency Department. Ann Emerg Med 2019;73(2): 183–92.

6. Simpson SA, Joesch JM, West II, et al. Risk for physical restraint or seclusion in the psychiatric emergency service (PES). Gen Hosp Psychiatry 2014;36(1): 113–8.

7. Retsas AP. Survey findings describing the use of physical restraints in nursing homes in Victoria, Australia. Int J Nurs Stud 1998;35(3):184–91.

8. Chan TC, Vilke GM, Neuman T, et al. Restraint position and positional asphyxia. Ann Emerg Med 1997;30(5):578–86.

9. Gault TI, Gray SM, Vilke GM, et al. Are Oral Medications Effective in the Management of Acute Agitation? Journal of EM 2012;43(5):854–9.

10. Perkins J, Ho JD, Vilke GM, et al. American Academy of Emergency Medicine Position Statement: Safety of Droperidol Use in the Emergency Department. J Emerg Med 2015;49(1):91–7.

11. Khokhar MA, Rathbone J. Droperidol for psychosis-induced aggression or agitation. Cochrane Database Syst Rev 2016;12(12):CD002830.

12. Thomas H, Schwartz E, Petrilli R. Droperidol versus haloperidol for chemical restraint of agitated and combative patients. Ann Emerg Med 1992;21(4):407–13.

13. ACOG Committee on Practice Bulletins–Obstetrics. ACOG Practice Bulletin: Clinical management guidelines for obstetrician-gynecologists number 92, April 2008 (replaces practice bulletin number 87, November 2007). Use of psychiatric medications during pregnancy and lactation. Obstet Gynecol 2008;111(4):1001–20.

14. Zimbroff DL, Allen MH, Battaglia J, et al. Best clinical practice with ziprasidone IM: update after 2 years of experience. CNS Spectr 2005;10(9):1–15.

15. Gunasekara NS, Spencer CM, Keating GM. Spotlight on ziprasidone in schizophrenia and schizoaffective disorder. CNS Drugs 2002;16(9):645–52.

16. Martel ML, Driver BE, Miner JR, et al. Randomized Double-blind Trial of Intramuscular Droperidol, Ziprasidone, and Lorazepam for Acute Undifferentiated Agitation in the Emergency Department. Acad Emerg Med 2021;28(4):421–34.

17. Martel M, Sterzinger A, Miner J, et al. Management of acute undifferentiated agitation in the emergency department: a randomized double-blind trial of droperidol, ziprasidone, and midazolam [published correction appears in Acad Emerg Med. 2006 Feb;13(2):233. Acad Emerg Med 2005;12(12):1167–72.

18. Klein LR, Driver BE, Horton G, et al. Rescue Sedation When Treating Acute Agitation in the Emergency Department With Intramuscular Antipsychotics. J Emerg Med 2019;56(5):484–90.

19. Khorassani F, Saad M. Intravenous Olanzapine for the Management of Agitation: Review of the Literature. Ann Pharmacother 2019;53(8):853–9.

20. Rund DA, Ewing JD, Mitzel K, et al. The use of intramuscular benzodiazpines and antipsychotic agents in the treatment of acute agtitation or violence in the emergency department. J Emerg Med 2006;31(3):317–24.

21. Mauri MC, Paletta S, Maffini M, et al. Clinical pharmacology of atypical antipsychotics: an update. EXCLI J 2014;13:1163–91.

22. Mancuso CE, Tanzi MG, Gabay M. Paradoxical reactions to benzodiazepines: literature review and treatment options. Pharmacotherapy 2004;24(9):1177–85.

23. Nobay F, Simon BC, Levitt MA, et al. A prospective, double-blind, randomized trial of midazolam versus haloperidol versus lorazepam in the chemical restraint of violent and severely agitated patients. Acad Emerg Med 2004;11(7):744–9.

24. Chan EW, Taylor DM, Knott JC, et al. Intravenous droperidol or olanzapine as an adjunct to midazolam for the acutely agitated patient: a multicenter, randomized, double-blind, placebo-controlled clinical trial. Ann Emerg Med 2013;61(1):72–81.

25. D Whitledge J, Fox ER, Mazer-Amirshahi M. Benzodiazepine Shortages: A Recurrent Challenge in Need of a Solution [published online ahead of print, 2022 Nov 21]. J Med Toxicol 2022. https://doi.org/10.1007/s13181-022-00917-z.

26. Riddell J, Tran A, Bengiamin R, et al. Ketamine as a first-line treatment for severely agitated emergency department patients. Am J Emerg Med 2017; 35(7):1000–4.

27. Barbic D, Andolfatto G, Grunau B, et al. Rapid Agitation Control With Ketamine in the Emergency Department: A Blinded, Randomized Controlled Trial. Ann Emerg Med 2021;78(6):788–95.

28. Lin J, Figuerado Y, Montgomery A, et al. Efficacy of ketamine for initial control of acute agitation in the emergency department: A randomized study. Am J Emerg Med 2021;44:306–11.

29. Strayer RJ, Nelson LS. Adverse events associated with ketamine for procedural sedation in adults [published correction appears in Am J Emerg Med. 2009 May;27(4):512. Am J Emerg Med 2008;26(9):985–1028.

30. Lahti AC, Koffel B, LaPorte D, et al. Subanesthetic doses of ketamine stimulate psychosis in schizophrenia. Neuropsychopharmacology 1995;13(1):9–19.

31. Zun LS. Evidence-Based Review of Pharmacotherapy for Acute Agitation. Part 1: Onset of Efficacy. J Emerg Med 2018;54(3):364–74.

32. Muir-Cochrane E, Oster C, Gerace A, et al. The effectiveness of chemical restraint in managing acute agitation and aggression: A systematic review of randomized controlled trials. Int J Ment Health Nurs 2020;29(2):110–26.

33. Klein LR, Driver BE, Miner JR, et al. Intramuscular Midazolam, Olanzapine, Ziprasidone, or Haloperidol for Treating Acute Agitation in the Emergency Department. Ann Emerg Med 2018;72(4):374–85.

34. Calver L, Drinkwater V, Gupta R, et al. Droperidol v. haloperidol for sedation of aggressive behaviour in acute mental health: randomised controlled trial. Br J Psychiatry 2015;206(3):223–8.

35. Battaglia J, Moss S, Rush J, et al. Haloperidol, lorazepam, or both for psychotic agitation? A multicenter, prospective, double-blind, emergency department study. Am J Emerg Med 1997;15(4):335–40.

36. Bieniek SA, Ownby RL, Penalver A, et al. A double-blind study of lorazepam versus the combination of haloperidol and lorazepam in managing agitation. Pharmacotherapy 1998;18(1):57–62.

37. Hui D, Frisbee-Hume S, Wilson A, et al. Effect of Lorazepam With Haloperidol vs Haloperidol Alone on Agitated Delirium in Patients With Advanced Cancer Receiving Palliative Care: A Randomized Clinical Trial. JAMA 2017;318(11): 1047–56.

38. Taylor DM, Yap CYL, Knott JC, et al. Midazolam-Droperidol, Droperidol, or Olanzapine for Acute Agitation: A Randomized Clinical Trial. Ann Emerg Med 2017; 69(3):318–26.e1.

39. Thiemann P, Roy D, Huecker M, et al. Prospective study of haloperidol plus lorazepam versus droperidol plus midazolam for the treatment of acute agitation in the emergency department. Am J Emerg Med 2022;55:76–81.
40. Jeffers T, Darling B, Edwards C, et al. Efficacy of Combination Haloperidol, Lorazepam, and Diphenhydramine vs. Combination Haloperidol and Lorazepam in the Treatment of Acute Agitation: A Multicenter Retrospective Cohort Study. J Emerg Med 2022;62(4):516–23.
41. Pittsenbarger ZE, Mannix R. Trends in pediatric visits to the emergency department for psychiatric illnesses. Acad Emerg Med 2014;21(1):25–30.
42. Kalb LG, Stapp EK, Ballard ED, et al. Trends in Psychiatric Emergency Department Visits Among Youth and Young Adults in the US. Pediatrics 2019;143(4): e20182192.
43. Grupp-Phelan J, Harman JS, Kelleher KJ. Trends in mental health and chronic condition visits by children presenting for care at U.S. emergency departments. Public Health Rep 2007;122(1):55–61.
44. Santillanes G, Gerson RS. Special Considerations in the Pediatric Psychiatric Population. Psychiatr Clin North Am 2017;40(3):463–73.
45. Department of Health and Human Services. Condition of participation: patient's rights. Fed Regist 2006;482:71426–8.
46. Rodriguez-Cabezas L, Clark C. Psychiatric emergencies in pregnancy and postpartum. Clin Obstet Gynecol 2018;61(3):615–27.
47. Aftab A, Shah AA. Behavioral emergencies: special considerations in the pregnant patient. Psychiatr Clin North Am 2017;40(3):435–48.
48. Iqbal MM, Aneja A, Rahman A, et al. The potential risks of commonly prescribed antipsychotics: during pregnancy and lactation. Psychiatry (Edgmont) 2005;2(8): 36–44.
49. Kulkarni J, Storch A, Baraniuk A, et al. Antipsychotic use in pregnancy. Expert Opin Pharmacother 2015;16(9):1335–45.
50. Allen MH, Currier GW, Carpenter D, et al. Expert Consensus Panel for Behavioral Emergencies 2005. The expert consensus guideline series. Treatment of behavioral emergencies 2005. J Psychiatr Pract 2005;11(Suppl 1):5–112.
51. Shenvi C, Kennedy M, Austin CA, et al. Managing Delirium and Agitation in the Older Emergency Department Patient: The ADEPT Tool. Ann Emerg Med 2020; 75(2):136–45.
52. By the American Geriatrics Society 2015 Beers Criteria Update Expert Panel. American Geriatrics Society 2015 Updated Beers Criteria for Potentially Inappropriate Medication Use in Older Adults. J Am Geriatr Soc 2015;63(11):2227–46.
53. Gastmans C, Milisen K. Use of physical restraint in nursing homes: clinical-ethical considerations. J Med Ethics 2006;32(3):148–52.
54. Frueh BC, Knapp RG, Cusack KJ, et al. Patients' reports of traumatic or harmful experiences within the psychiatric setting. Psychiatr Serv 2005;56(9):1123–33.

Emergency Department Care of the Patient with Suicidal or Homicidal Symptoms

Chadd K. Kraus, DO, DrPH[a,b,]*, James Ferry, DO[c]

KEYWORDS

- Emergency department • Mental illness • Psychiatric illness • Suicidality
- Homicidally • Psychiatric boarding • Involuntary commitment

KEY POINTS

- Patients presenting to the emergency department (ED) with suicidality or homicidally should undergo a thorough medical screening examination to determine whether they have an emergency medical condition that requires timely intervention, should be stabilized in a timely manner, and should have treatment, including hospitalization for psychiatric care, initiated to ensure the safety of the patient and others, including ED staff.
- The needs of patients presenting to the ED are frequently mismatched to available resources, creating unique challenges for the emergency physician and care team in the ED.
- Determining appropriate disposition, whether inpatient or outpatient, requires a thorough understanding of local laws and regulations, as well as consideration of available resources and the patient's unique circumstances and needs.

INTRODUCTION

The demand for mental health and psychiatric care has increased exponentially over the past several decades with a 44 percent increase in emergency department (ED) visits for psychiatric and behavioral health concerns since 2006.[1] This trend was exacerbated during the COVID-19 pandemic. Among youth and adolescents, there has been nearly a 30 percent increase in psychiatric ED visits in recent years.[2] These trends were exacerbated during the COVID-19 pandemic.[3,4]

EDs are frequently utilized by individuals experiencing a mental health crisis. Individuals with psychiatric and behavioral health conditions are five times more likely to be frequent ED users than individuals without mental health concerns.[5,6] Nearly 1 in 10 visits to EDs in the United States involve a psychiatric or substance-use related

[a] Department of Emergency and Hospital Medicine, Lehigh Valley Health Network, Allentown, PA, USA; [b] University of South Florida Morsani College of Medicine; [c] Department of Emergency Medicine, Geisinger, Danville, Pennsylvania, USA
* Corresponding author. University of South Florida Morsani College of Medicine.
E-mail address: chaddkraus@gmail.com

Emerg Med Clin N Am 42 (2024) 31–40
https://doi.org/10.1016/j.emc.2023.06.021
0733-8627/24/© 2023 Elsevier Inc. All rights reserved.

emed.theclinics.com

diagnosis.[7] Suicide is the 10th leading cause of death in the United States and the second leading cause of death among those ages 15 to 24 years.[8] An index visit to the ED with self-harm or suicidal ideation is associated with a significantly higher risk of suicide and other mortality during the year after ED presentation.[9,10] Approximately 10 percent of individuals who die by suicide, and 9 percent who die by homicide visit an ED within 6 weeks prior to death.[11] Particularly among patients presenting with suicidal ideation, dual diagnosis of substance use psychiatric diagnoses are common, and often involve more than one substance.[12] Patients with psychiatric and behavioral health disorders often have a range of chronic physical illness as well.[6] While most patients present voluntarily for evaluation, some are brought to the ED by family, emergency medical services (EMS), police, behavioral health crisis workers, or by other means. In other cases, patients may present for non-mental illness related complaints only to be found to have significant psychiatric symptoms.

The objective of this review is to provide an overview of the evaluation, stabilization, treatment, and disposition of patients with acute suicidal or homicidal symptoms presenting to the ED. This includes a high-level discussion of the voluntary and involuntary psychiatric evaluation process. Specific rules pertaining to the process of voluntary and involuntary examination and treatment vary by state and/or county and local laws regulations that should be understood to govern and guide decisions.

INITIAL EVALUATION

As with all patients in the ED, the immediate identification and stabilization of threats to a patient's life, limb, or vision are of primary concern in those presenting with behavioral health and psychiatric symptoms. A thorough history and physical examination are necessary in the initial evaluation. In alert, adult patients presenting to the ED with acute psychiatric symptoms, routine laboratory testing has little clinical utility and should not be ordered.[13–15] If history or physical examination raises concern for or confirms a toxic ingestion of a drug or other substance, reveals alcohol intoxication, uncovers a traumatic injury, or has other features that suggest an emergency medical condition in addition to the acute psychiatric symptom(s), then additional diagnostic evaluation might be warranted.

The triage process in many EDs includes a general question about mental health, often specifically about suicidality.[16] There are multiple validated suicide screening tools, including the Ask Suicide-Screening Questions (ASQ), the Suicide Behavior Questionnaire-Revised (SBQ-R), the Columbia Suicide Severity Rating Scale (C-SSRS), the Public Health Questionnaire-9 (PHQ-9), and the Patient Safety Screener-3 (PSS-3). The unique environment of the ED, and the need for rapid, timely assessment and determination of patients at risk for suicide limits the application of some of these tools in the initial evaluation of a patient. The "Ask Suicide-Screening Questions" (ASQ), a set of 4 questions that takes approximately 20 seconds to administer, has been successfully used in the ED to identify patients at risk for suicide.[17,18] ASQ can be used for patients of all ages in the ED.[18]

EPs can address immediate safety concerns, stabilize patients, and facilitate inpatient hospitalization, but may lack the robust resources to initiate additional treatments and link patients to necessary outpatient care. There is frequently a lack of psychiatric and behavioral health resources for the ED team to utilize in caring for patients with psychiatric symptoms, and along with these resource limitations, patients can have negative experiences related to the environmental stimuli characteristic of an ED.[19] These same patients can have prolonged ED boarding times, in many cases up to 24 hours or longer, awaiting admission or transfer to inpatient psychiatric care.

Patients with psychiatric and behavioral health needs who are boarding in the ED are at increased risk of adverse events including increased agitation, chemical or physical sedation, verbal and physical assaults on ED staff, and additional restrictions on patient movement while in the ED (eg, being locked in a treatment room).[20] These risks increase with longer boarding times.[20] ED boarding of patients in need of psychiatric care also increases the inpatient hospital length of stay for those patients.[21]

Patients with acute behavioral health and psychiatric crises represent a special population of patients requiring emergency care. The needs of these patients are frequently mismatched to available resources, creating unique challenges for the emergency physician and care team in the ED. However, these patients are often unable to receive the timely care that they require, particularly for disposition to either an inpatient psychiatric unit or for medication and therapeutic interventions necessary for acute stabilization followed by transition to comprehensive and continuing outpatient treatment.

Diagnostic and Treatment Considerations

Patients with acute psychiatric and behavioral health presentations must be stabilized, including if necessary, pharmacologic sedation and, in extreme cases, physical restraint to protect patients and others. Patients who are physically restrained and involuntarily committed to the hospital often cite a lack of understanding from and poor communication with the health care team regarding decision about physical restraint.[22,23] The safety of the patient and ED staff should be the first priority throughout the ED stay.

The landmark 1974 ruling by the California Supreme Court, Tarasoff v. Regents of the University of California, established the precedent that health care professionals have a duty to warn individuals who might be harmed by a patient who expresses intent to harm that individual.[24] Diagnostic and treatment considerations for patients with suicidal and homicidal patients should be personalized and framed within the context of by local and regional resources and impacted by existing laws and regulations governing local practice environments.

Multiple system-level approaches and innovations, including re-designing the physical space of the ED have been suggested to facilitate the disposition of patients presenting to EDs with the psychiatric and behavioral health conditions including suicidality and homicidality. For example, Emergency Psychiatric Assessment, Treatment, and Healing (EmPATH) units provide a space within the ED dedicated to patients with psychiatric symptoms as well as timely access to evaluation by a psychiatrist. Early results suggest that EmPATH units successfully reduce ED boarding and unnecessary admissions and help to establish post-ED care with a 60 percent improvement in 30-day follow-up.[25] Other alternative psychiatric emergency services programs such as the Boston Emergency Services Team (BEST) uses a multi-modal approach including specialized psychiatric EDs, a 24/7 hotline, psychiatric urgent care centers, and mobile crisis units, to reduce ED encounters by 12 percent.[26] Among youth patients with behavioral health needs, community-based mobile crisis services can reduce ED visits.[27]

Involuntary Commitment

Involuntary commitment for psychiatric symptoms is based on the legal principle of parens patriae. Parens patriae is the concept that the government or another authority has an obligation to protect those who are unable to protect themselves. Similarly, for patients with suicidal or homicidal thoughts, the health care team has the obligation to protect a patient who is a danger to themselves or others.

Involuntary commitment should be reserved for rare instances in which the patient is a risk to himself and does not have the capacity and is unable to consent or participate in initial treatment decisions that are intended to stabilize the patient and provide immediate protection to them. Emergency physicians should reserve involuntary commitment for those cases in which a patient with acute behavioral and psychiatric needs represents a danger to themselves or others and are unable to adequately recognize the severity of the acuity illness in a way that impedes their safe execution of self-care.[28] Specific laws and regulations related to involuntary hospitalization and treatment differ according to local jurisdiction. The emergency physician should be familiar with those local laws.

Involuntary commitment can result in a patient feeling coerced and can ultimately negatively impact the therapeutic relationship and outcome. Involuntary commitment can be reminiscent of historical models of indefinite inpatient hospitalizations in institutions that were primarily custodial and less focused on treatment and management of acute behavioral health and mental illness.[29]

The use of involuntary commitment should be based on traditional tenets of medical ethics, and to the degree possible, aimed to protect patient autonomy and self-determination. Barring immediate danger to self or others, the approach to disposition must focus on a least restrictive plan that incorporates a patient's informed consent. Disposition using involuntary treatment is ultimately aimed at improving the patient's health to restore autonomy.[30]

Voluntary examination and treatment

A patient voluntarily presenting for psychiatric evaluation can authorize their own treatment. An authorization is a signed document that outlines the pertinent findings on interview and physical examination as well as the proposed treatment and interventions. It is a form of informed consent for treatment. A patient may withdraw from this agreement at any time by giving written notice, however release can be delayed up to 72 hours provided delayed release was specified in the initial voluntary agreement. If a patient who agrees to voluntary hospitalization for psychiatric treatment decides later that they do not want to be hospitalized, a reassessment of their immediate risks to self and others should be completed. The patient might be appropriate for discharge, and if they are not and remain at risk for self-harm or harm to others, it might be necessary to proceed with involuntary admission.

The signing of a voluntary treatment agreement does not necessitate inpatient hospitalization and the patient can subsequently be discharged if hospitalization is not found to be necessary. Typically, this determination is made by the psychiatrist and members of the behavioral health team after interviewing the patient, however in some cases the determination might be made by the emergency physician. It should be noted that in cases of very minor psychiatric symptoms, an evaluation can be completed with only verbal authorization by the patient. However, if further evaluation is deemed necessary after initial evaluation of a patient, written authorization for voluntary examination and treatment should be obtained.

There are some states that allow patients under the age of 18 to sign an agreement for voluntary evaluation. As noted above regulations vary by state and this is particularly true for how minors are handled. For instance, in some states, such as Pennsylvania, a patient aged 14 or greater can volunteer for inpatient treatment. However, if a patient is 14 to 17 years of age and not emancipated, a voluntary commitment can be signed by the parent or legal guardian if the patient is not willing to do so. If a patient is under the age of 14, an agreement for voluntary evaluation and treatment can only be signed by the patient's parent or legal guardian.

Prior to hospitalization, a patient must be deemed medically appropriate for inpatient psychiatric hospitalization. As previously described, this medical evaluation usually involves a history and physical examination and depending on specific circumstances might involve additional diagnostic testing. Patients under voluntary treatment may not be transferred from one facility to another without their consent. If a patient is a minor (and not emancipated) transfer consent must be obtained from the parent or legal guardian regardless of who signed the voluntary treatment agreement (ie, transfer agreements cannot be signed by unemancipated minors).

Involuntary examination and treatment

A patient presenting involuntarily to the ED due to a mental health crisis may be made subject to involuntary emergency examination and treatment. If a person is believed to be severely incapacitated because of mental illness to the extent that they can reasonably be considered a risk to themself, a risk to others, or to lack decision-making capacity, they can be subject to involuntary examination, treatment, and hospitalization.

A petition for involuntary examination and treatment can be made by anyone with familiarity with the patient that has observed behavior concerning for significant mental illness or disability. Most often this person is a family member, partner, neighbor, law enforcement, or an emergency physician. Once a petition is made, the patient must be made aware of their rights. Rights are typically read by a designee of the county, but this process can vary based on state and county. An attempt must be made to make a patient aware of their rights regardless of their perceived capacity to understand them. However, if a patient lacks the ability to understand their rights due to their mental illness, this does not preclude them from involuntary examination and treatment. Once a petition is made and rights are read, a patient can be interviewed and examined by the emergency physician who, in many circumstances, will consult a psychiatrist for recommendations. If the patient is deemed unfit for discharge due to mental illness, and inappropriate or unwilling to agree to voluntary hospitalization, it would then be suitable to "uphold" a petition for involuntary hospitalization and treatment. Petitions for involuntary examination and treatment can only be upheld by a physician. Involuntary commitment cannot exceed 120 hours without further legal steps that are beyond the scope of this review and are typically handled by psychiatric facility staff.

Safety planning

What is it? Safety planning is a collaborative process between a patient identified as having increased risk for suicide and the medical professional. The goal of safety planning is to reduce risk of suicide. Safety planning attempts to achieve suicide risk reduction by identifying the patient's strengths and unique resources to increase safety and reduce risky behavior. The medical professional is most often a therapist, psychiatrist, or emergency physician but other medical professionals are not excluded.[31]

Who should have it? Safety planning should be performed on all patients who are deemed appropriate for discharge from a health care setting, but also have risk factors consistent with increased risk for suicide. A 2018 study revealed that threshold for safety planning varies greatly by facility, from performing safety planning with all patients at one end of the spectrum to only completing safety planning with patients that both have a history of suicide and are currently having suicidal thoughts.[31] While it is impractical to perform safety planning on all patients, it is advisable to capture as many patients as possible given the demonstrated reduction of suicide attempt in patients who have had safety planning completed.

How should it be done? The basic components of safety planning are as follows:

1. Identify warning signs or triggers that indicate suicide ideation is likely to occur
2. List internal coping strategies for use when those triggers occur or when experiencing suicide ideation
3. List social contacts for further distraction or social locations that may provide distraction
4. List supportive contacts along with contact information
5. List emergency resources (eg, therapist phone numbers, hotlines, local hospital emergency department locations)
6. Take steps to ensure the safety of the home environment that minimize the patient's ability to act on suicidal thoughts or urges (limiting/removing access to firearms, knives, medications)[32]

Note: If a patient is not already established with a psychiatrist at the time of safety planning, a referral should be made.

AFTER PLAN IS DEVELOPED: ASSESS, DISCUSS, EVALUATE, AND REVIEW

Assess–Review the completed safety plan with the patient to identify and clarify any areas of confusion and to identify and address any barriers to utilizing the plan in its current form.

Discuss–Clarify with the patient where they will keep the safety plan so to ensure it will be available to them in the event of a crisis.

Evaluate–Confirm that the patient understands the safety plan and that they will be able to utilize it on their own or with the assistance of another person who can reasonably be assumed to be available to them.

Review–The safety plan can evolve over time as needs change. It should be reviewed periodically and updated as appropriate.

DISPOSITION

Patients presenting to the ED with suicidal or homicidal thoughts might be hospitalized voluntarily or involuntarily as described above, or they might be discharged with close outpatient follow-up. Disposition of patients with suicidal or homicidal thoughts from the ED should be personalized. Admission and discharge can both be delayed by barriers including bed availability, transportation, and social factors such as family support.[33] Achieving the most appropriate disposition for an individual patient requires a team and interdisciplinary approach including case management.

Patients presenting to the ED for psychiatric symptoms might express active suicidality, describing a specific plan, or might experience passive suicidality, or suicidal thoughts without a plan. Both situations can be dangerous and conversely, in some instances, outpatient follow-up might be appropriate. There are currently no validated risk assessment and stratification tools to identify patients with suicidal ideation who are safe for discharge from the ED. The preferred approach to determining risk in these patients is a holistic approach that includes a combination of "appropriate psychiatric assessment, good clinical judgment, [and] taking patient, family, and community factors into account."[15] Patients presenting to the ED with suicidal or homicidal thoughts might be able to be safely discharged for outpatient management.

Linkage to outpatient care is critically important to providing care for patients with suicidality or homicidality in the ED. At least one study estimated 40 percent of patients received inadequate or no outpatient care following an ED visit for a psychiatric complaint.[34] In addition to reducing return visits to the ED, timely follow-up with outpatient psychiatric services reduces risk of death by suicide following inpatient psychiatric hospitalization.[35] When follow-up care is available within 30 days of discharge from a psychiatric hospitalization, the risk of readmission is reduced.[36] Barriers to outpatient follow-up include patients' complex health and social circumstances, establishing relationships with outpatient providers, and availability and coordination of care between the ED and outpatient settings.[37]

It is critically important to address these needs for all patients presenting to the ED, including special populations such as pediatric and geriatric patients. Additionally, populations such as those persons with developmental delays or autism spectrum disorders have additional specific needs and can require special approaches to best meet their needs comprehensively. For the discussion herein, these patients will not be considered separately. More than 1 in 4 children who are seen in the emergency department for a mental health visit return within 6 months, whereas timely outpatient follow-up within 30 days decreased the risk of return within 5 days of the index ED visits by 26 percent.[38] However, only about half of children have access to a follow-up appointment within 30 days of their index ED visit.[38]

Consideration should be made for how the time-limited encounter in the ED of an acute exacerbation of illness might impact, positively or negatively, the patient's overall mental health, including future risk for suicidality.[39] Similar to the impact of ED evaluation and management of other conditions (eg, missed myocardial infarction, delayed treatment for stroke, delayed diagnosis or treatment in sepsis), the acute management of patients with behavioral health conditions can have lasting impacts. As such, the emergency physician should consider the ED encounter in the context of the patient's broader needs in behavioral health. As community-based psychiatric resources continue to be strained and, in some areas, unavailable, the ED will continue to play an increasing role in the spectrum of care of this vulnerable population of patients.

SUMMARY

Patients presenting to the ED with acute psychiatric and behavioral health concerns require the same timely, thorough, and quality care as other patients presenting to the ED. This population of patients must be evaluated, treated, and hospitalized or discharged with outpatient follow-up often amid inadequate clinical and system resources to provide that care in the ED. Future work in this area includes assessments of innovations that optimize the availability of psychiatric resources both in and outside of the ED.

CLINICS CARE POINTS

- Timely evaluation is required to initiate necessary stabilization and ensure patient and ED staff safety.
- Patient autonomy should be persevered, focusing on a least restrictive approach while in the ED and while developing a treatment and disposition plan.
- Local laws and regulations should be considered in disposition decisions, including voluntary and involuntary hospitalization.
- Discharged patients should be linked to outpatient follow-up care to be completed as soon as possible.

DISCLOSURES

Dr C.K. Kraus and Dr J. Ferry have no financial or other conflicts of interest to disclose related to this work.

REFERENCES

1. Moore B, Stocks C, Owens PL. Trends in emergency department visits, 2006–2014. HCUP Statistical Brief #227. Washington, DC, USA: Agency for Healthcare Research and Quality (AHRQ); 2017.
2. Kalb LG, Stapp EK, Ballard ED, et al. Trends in psychiatric emergency department visits among youth and young adults in the US. Pediatrics 2019;143(4): e20182192.
3. Holland KM, Jones C, Vivolo-Kantor AM, et al. Trends in US emergency department visits for mental health, overdose, and violence outcomes before and during the COVID-19 pandemic. JAMA Psychiatr 2021;78(4):372–9.
4. Leeb RT, Bitsko RH, Radhakrishnan L, et al. Centers for disease control and prevention (CDC). Mental health-related emergency department visits among children aged <18 years during the COVID-19 pandemic – United States, January 1 – October 17, 2020. MMWR Morb Mortal Wkly Rep 2020;69(45):1675–80.
5. Brennan JJ, Chan TC, Hsia RY, et al. Emergency department utilization among frequent users with psychiatric visits. Acad Emerg Med 2014;21:1015–22.
6. Gentil L, Grenier G, Meng X, et al. Impact of co-occurring mental disorders and chronic physical illnesses on frequency of emergency department use and hospitalization for mental health reasons. Front Psychiatry 2021;12:735005.
7. Theriault KM, Rosenheck RA, Rhee TG. Increasing emergency department visits for mental health conditions in the United States. J Clin Psychiatry 2020;81(5): 20m13241.
8. Borecky A, Thomsen C, Dubov A. Reweighing the ethical tradeoffs in the involuntary hospitalization of suicidal patients. Am J Bioeth 2019;19(10):71–83.
9. Goldman-Mellor S, Offson M, Lidon-Moyano C, et al. Association of suicide and other mortality with emergency department presentation. JAMA Netw Open 2019; 2(12):e1917571.
10. Olfson M, Gao YN, Xie M, et al. Suicide risk among adults with mental health emergency department visits with and without suicidal symptoms. J Clin Psychiatry 2021;82(6):20m13833.
11. Cerel J, Singleton MD, Brown MM, et al. Emergency department visits prior to suicide and homicide: linking statewide surveillance systems. Crisis 2016; 37(1):5–12.
12. Tadros A, Sharon M, Crum M, et al. Coexistence of substance abuse among emergency department patients presenting with suicidal ideation. BioMed Res Int 2020;746701.
13. Korn CS, Currier GW, Henderson SO. "Medical Clearance" of psychiatric patients without medical complaints in the emergency department. J Emerg Med 2000; 18(2):173–6.
14. Conigliaro A, Benabbas R, Schnitzer E, et al. Protocolized laboratory screening for the medical clearance of psychiatric patients in the emergency department: a systematic review. Acad Emerg Med 2018;25:566–76.
15. Clinical Policies Subcommittee (Writing Committee) on the Adult Psychiatric Patient, Nazarian DJ, Broder JS, Thiessen MEW, et al. Clinical policy: critical issues in the diagnosis and management of the adult psychiatric patient in the

emergency department. American College of Emergency Physicians Ann Emerg Med 2017;69(4):480–98.

16. Wolf LA, Perhats C, Delao AM, et al. Assessing for occult suicidality at triage: experiences of emergency nurses. J Emerg Nurs 2018;44(5):491–8.

17. Horowitz LM, Bridge JA, Teach SJ, et al. Ask suicide-screening questions (ASQ). Arch Pediatr Adolesc Med 2012;166(12):1170–6.

18. National Institute of Mental Health. Ask Suicide-Screening (ASQ)Toolkit. Available online at: https://www.nimh.nih.gov/research/research-conducted-at-nimh/asq-toolkit-materials. (Last accessed February 28, 2023).

19. Hoge MA, Vanderploeg J, Paris M Jr, et al. Emergency department use by children and youth with mental health conditions: a health equity agenda. Community Ment Health J 2022;58(7):1225–39.

20. Major D, Rittenbach K, MacMaster F, et al. Exploring the experience of boarded psychiatric patients in adult emergency departments. BMC Psychiatry 2021; 21(1):473.

21. Lane DJ, Roberts L, Currie S, et al. Association of emergency department times on hospital length of stay for patients with psychiatric illness. Emerg Med J 2022; 39(7):494–500.

22. Wong AH, Ray JM, Rosenberg A, et al. Experiences of individuals who were physically restrained in the emergency department. JAMA Netw Open 2020;3: e1919381.

23. Navas C, Wells L, Bartels SA, et al. Patient and provider perspectives on emergency department care experiences among people with mental health concerns. Healthcare (Basel) 2022;10(7):1297.

24. Tarasoff v. Regents of University of California (1974). Available online at: https://caselaw.findlaw.com/ca-supreme-court/1829929.html. (Last accessed, February 26, 2023).

25. Kim AK, Vakkalanka JP, Van Heukelom P, et al. Emergency psychiatric assessment, treatment, and healing (EmPATH) unit decreases hospital admission for patients presenting with suicidal ideation in rural America. Acad Emerg Med 2022; 29(2):142–9.

26. Oblath R, Herrera CN, Ware LPO, et al. Long-term trends in psychiatric emergency services delivered by the Boston Emergency Services Team. Community Ment Health J 2023;59(2):370–80.

27. Fendrich M, Ives M, Kurz B, et al. Impact of mobile crisis services on emergency department use among youths with behavioral health service needs. Psychiatr Serv 2019;70(10):881–7.

28. Testa M, West SG. Civil commitment in the United States. Psychiatry (Edgmont) 2010;7(10):30.

29. Saya A, Brugnoli C, Piazzi G, et al. Criteria, procedures, and future prospects of involuntary treatment in psychiatry around the world. A Narrative Review 2019; 10:271.

30. Sjöstrand M, Sandman L, Karlsson P, et al. Ethical deliberations about involuntary treatment: interviews with Swedish psychiatrists. BMC Med Ethics 2015;16(1):37.

31. Moscardini EH, Hill RM, Dodd CG, et al. Suicide safety planning: clinician training, comfort, and safety plan utilization. Int J Environ Res Publ Health 2020;17(18):6444.

32. Suicide Prevention Resource Center. Safety Planning Guide: A Quick Guide for Clinicians. Available Online at: https://www.sprc.org/resources-programs/safety-planning-guide-quick-guide-clinicians. (Last accessed January 6, 2023).

33. Kraft CM, Morea P, Teresi B, et al. Characteristics, clinical care, and disposition barriers for mental health patients boarding in the emergency department. Am J Emerg Med 2021;46:550–5.
34. Gabet M, Cao Z, Fleury M-J. Profiles, correlates and outcome among patients experiencing an onset of mental disorder based on outpatient care received following index emergency department visits. Can J Psychiatry 2022;67(10): 787–801.
35. Fontanella CA, Warner LA, Steelesmith DL, et al. Association of timely outpatient mental health services for youths after psychiatric hospitalization with risk of death by suicide. JAMA Netw Open 2020;3(8):e2012887.
36. Fleury M-J, Gentil L, Grenier G, et al. The impact of 90-day physician follow-up care on the risk of readmission following a psychiatric hospitalization. Adm Policy Ment Health 2022;49(6):1047–59.
37. Walker ER, Fukuda J, McMonigle M, et al. A qualitative study of barriers and facilitators to transitions from the emergency department to outpatient mental health care. Psychiatr Serv 2021;72(11):1311–9.
38. Hoffmann JA, Krass P, Rodean J, et al. Follow-up after pediatric mental health emergency visits. Pediatrics 2023;151(3). e2022057383.
39. Xu Z, Muller M, Lay B, et al. Involuntary hospitalization, stigma stress, and suicidality: a longitudinal study. Soc Psychiatry Psychiatr Epidemiol 2018;53(3): 309–12.

Hyperactive Delirium with Severe Agitation

Brian Springer, MD

KEYWORDS

- Excited delirium • Hyperactive delirium with severe agitation • Altered mental status
- In-custody deaths • Restraint • Catecholamine surge • Hyperadrenergic state
- Hyperthermia

KEY POINTS

- Hyperactive delirium with severe agitation is a clinical syndrome of altered mental status, psychomotor agitation, and a hyperadrenergic state.
- Hyperactive delirium most often results from sympathomimetic abuse, psychiatric disease, sedative-hypnotic withdrawal, and metabolic derangements.
- Although the underlying pathophysiology remains undetermined and likely highly variable, it is postulated that high levels of endogenous catecholamines related to exertion and stress, combined with concomitant stimulant abuse plus physical struggle or restraint, result in hypoxia, hyperkalemia, acidosis, and autonomic dysfunction.
- Patients suffering from hyperactive delirium can go from a hyperdynamic and combative state to periarrest or perimortem with little to no warning.
- Although several cases of in-custody death have resulted in scrutiny of rapid sedation of severely agitated patients, the use of benzodiazepines, antipsychotics, or ketamine in the prehospital or ED setting is effective and safe, with the risk of airway loss and decompensation being most likely secondary to coingestions and the underlying disease state.

BACKGROUND AND CONTROVERSIES

The syndrome of delirium with severe agitation was first described in the 1800s, and over the last 200 years has been referred to by multiple names. These include Bell mania, exhaustive mania, lethal catatonia, agitated delirium, excited delirium syndrome (ExDS), and most recently hyperactive delirium with severe agitation. In the 1970s the presentation became associated with acute cocaine intoxication and psychosis, sometimes through intentional ingestion but more often from accidental overdose when ingested packets broke open in the bodies of smugglers. Seizures, coma, respiratory failure, and death often followed.[1,2] The contemporary term, excited delirium, was first described in the modern literature in 1985 as the sudden onset

Division of Tactical Emergency Medicine, Department of Emergency Medicine, Wright State University, 2555 University Boulevard, Suite 110, Fairborn, OH 45324, USA
E-mail address: brian.springer@wright.edu

Emerg Med Clin N Am 42 (2024) 41–52
https://doi.org/10.1016/j.emc.2023.06.011
0733-8627/24/© 2023 Elsevier Inc. All rights reserved.

emed.theclinics.com

of bizarre, paranoid, and violent behavior, associated with unexpected physical strength and hyperthermia. Fatal collapse occurred within minutes to hours of restraint. Again, most cases were reported as linked to stimulant drug intoxication, such as cocaine (predominantly), methamphetamine, and phencyclidine. In some cases, psychiatric or systemic illness were believed to be contributing factors.[2] Many of these cases involved a struggle with law enforcement, including physical, chemical, or electrical control measures. Autopsy usually failed to yield a definitive cause of death. Currently, there are multiple definitions of excited delirium, none of which is universally recognized, and many based on variable criteria.[3] As a result, it remains a clinically based syndrome, prone to much subjectivity in the scientific literature. It has been argued that excited delirium is not a valid diagnosis, and that the term is used as a means of deflecting the investigation of in-custody deaths away from the actions of law enforcement personnel, with the goal of exonerating law enforcement and covering up police brutality.[4,5] Excited delirium and ExDS are not recognized as exact diagnoses in the International Classification of Diseases-10. A patient may be diagnosed with cocaine delirium or delirium from a specific or unspecified stimulant or other psychoactive substance, but not with the specific syndrome.

In 2009, the American College of Emergency Physicians (ACEP) published the White Paper Report on Excited Delirium Syndrome.[6] The purpose of the review behind the white paper was three-fold: determine the existence (or not) of ExDS as a disease entity, determine the characteristics that help identify the presentation of excited delirium and the risk of death, and look at current and emerging methods of control and treatment. The task force behind the paper proposed a definition based on a syndromic approach, where ExDS is identified by the presence of distinctive clinical and behavioral criteria that is recognized in the premortem state. They noted that although potentially fatal, in some cases it is amenable to early therapeutic interventions. The syndrome is characterized by delirium, agitation, and hyperadrenergic autonomic dysfunction, often in the setting of acute on chronic substance abuse or severe mental illness. The features recommended by the White Paper task force as diagnostic for ExDS are neither consistently seen in other studies nor mandatory for ExDS to be present; additionally, the criteria are not seen with the same frequency between studies and case series.[3]

The 2009 White Paper report has been the subject of considerable controversy. It was published before ACEP established its current conflict-of-interest policy, and it was noted that authors had financial interest in law enforcement less-lethal technology, whose use has been associated with in-custody deaths. Several authors have called for an end of the use of the term ExDS, especially as a cause of in-custody death. They believe that the term, along with associated use of ketamine and other pharmacologic agents, are used as justification for excessive police force, and that the term is disproportionately cited when Black and Brown men die while in police custody.[7–10] A policy adopted in 2021 by the American Medical Association at their House of Delegates meeting[7]

- Confirms the American Medical Association stance that current evidence does not support "excited delirium" as an official diagnosis, and opposes its use until a clear set of diagnostic criteria has been established
- Denounces "excited delirium" as a sole justification for law enforcement use of excessive force
- Underscores the importance of emergency physician–led oversight of medical emergencies in the field

- Opposes the use of sedative/hypnotic and dissociative drugs, including ketamine, as an intervention for an agitated individual in a law enforcement setting, without a legitimate medical reason
- Recognizes the risk that sedative/hypnotic and dissociative drugs have in relation to an individual's age, underlying medical conditions, and potential drug interactions when used outside of a hospital setting by a nonphysician

In response to these ongoing controversies, ACEP created a task force to answer the questions surrounding the initial management of patients presenting with severe agitation, and released their report in 2021.[11] Given the charged nature of the term ExDS, the authors instead elected to use the term "hyperactive delirium with severe agitation." The authors acknowledge that the task force report is not meant to refute the findings of the White Paper. In fact, the report features an extended overview of definition, epidemiology, and pathophysiology of ExDS. They acknowledge the weaknesses in the literature and controversy surrounding the definition, and ultimately group management under the term hyperactive delirium. For the purposes of this paper, the terms "hyperactive delirium with severe agitation," "hyperactive delirium," or simply "severe agitation" are used, with the understanding that ExDS is part of this clinical syndrome, and that the literature cited predominantly reflects the study of ExDS with its associated literature biases and controversies.

CLINICAL FEATURES

Without a specific cause or single anatomic feature, hyperactive delirium is best described by its common clinical presentations and usual course. These are highly subjective, with the literature often depending on an a priori definition of ExDS or similar that lacks clearly defined objective criteria.[11] The consistent clinical prerequisites are a condition of altered mental status (disorientation, impaired judgment and thought, disruptions in perception, psychomotor skills, and behavior), psychomotor agitation, and a hyperadrenergic state. Given the varied underlying medical insults that can generate hyperactive delirium, there is variation in the presenting symptom cluster. It is the combination of delirium, psychomotor agitation, and physiologic excitation that differentiates hyperactive delirium from processes that result in delirium alone, or from individuals who are agitated and violent but not delirious.[6]

In the prehospital setting, the features most often associated with hyperactive delirium are

- Constant or near constant physical activity with a lack of tiring (sometimes perceived as "superhuman" strength)
- Increased/abnormal pain tolerance
- Tachypnea
- Diaphoresis
- Tactile hyperthermia
- Noncompliance/failure to respond to police presence

Other less common features include disrobing, nudity, or inappropriate clothing, and an unusual attraction to glass, mirrors, or other reflective surfaces.[6,12] Among a large Canadian cohort used to derive the previously mentioned features, subjects with three or more features were involved in 1 of every 11 use of force encounters, and individuals with six or more features were involved in 1 in 66 use of force encounters.[12] Most patients in the cohort did not die, countering opinion that "excited delirium" is a contrived condition to excuse improper procedure or excessive force. This also runs contrary to the older literature, where death was part of the definition.

This likely reflects publication bias from forensic physicians who were looking specifically at fatal cases.[3]

Patients who die tend to die suddenly, often following physical, chemical, or electrical control measures, and with no clear anatomic cause of death noted on autopsy.[6] Along with the clinical features mentioned previously, fatal cases include the following:

- Male gender
- Mean age mid-30s
- Destructive or bizarre behavior, including violence toward inanimate objects, that generate a call to police
- Suspected use of psychostimulants or history of psychostimulant abuse
- History of or suspected psychiatric illness
- Sudden cardiopulmonary collapse following a struggle and restraint, or shortly after a period of quiescence or "giving up"
- Inability to be resuscitated on scene, despite aggressive efforts

The differential diagnosis for hyperactive delirium covers a wide range of disease states associated with altered mental status. Hyperactive delirium commonly results from intoxication with cocaine, methamphetamine, and other stimulants. Clinical findings of sympathomimetic toxicity include tachycardia, tachypnea, hypertension, hyperthermia, and diaphoresis. Other physical findings include tremor, myoclonus, and lower extremity rigidity. Mental status changes include aggression, repetitive behaviors, hallucinations, and psychosis. Psychiatric disease, sedative-hypnotic withdrawal, and metabolic derangements are also associated with hyperactive delirium in patients without a history of sympathomimetic abuse.[11]

There are several specific disease states that may resemble hyperactive delirium and deserve mention.[4,6] Diabetic hypoglycemia may resemble intoxication and result in violent behaviors. Diagnosis is made rapidly with bedside glucose testing. Classic and exertional heat stroke may result in tactile hyperthermia and delirium and can occur with neuroleptic use in mental illness. A significantly elevated core temperature should prompt initiation of rapid cooling. Thyroid storm may result in hyperthermia and altered mental status, and thyroid function testing should be included in a comprehensive work-up. Serotonin syndrome and neuroleptic malignant syndrome are associated with mental status changes, neuromuscular hyperactivity, and autonomic hyperactivity, and may be difficult to differentiate from hyperactive delirium, and from each other (**Box 1**).

EPIDEMIOLOGY

With hyperactive delirium with severe agitation being a recently labeled condition, and with no standardized definition existing for ExDS, determining the exact incidence is not possible. The prevalence seems to vary widely based on the case definition and the context in which the episodes are described. Settings include emergency medical services (EMS) encounters, police encounters, in the emergency department (ED) or hospital, and forensic investigations. Forensic literature looks specifically at ExDS as a diagnosis of exclusion based on autopsy, with little documentation or discussion about survivors. It also demonstrates a high association with conducted energy weapon–related deaths and cocaine-related deaths. It is uncommon among EMS encounters as a whole, with severe cases requiring restraint documented in less than 2 cases per 10,000 advanced life support calls.[3,4]

Severe agitation is a common problem in EDs, although rates of presentation vary greatly, even among busy urban systems. Highest prevalence reported lies around

---

Box 1
Hyperactive delirium with severe agitation differential diagnosis

- Sympathomimetic toxidrome
  - Hypertension, tachycardia, mydriasis, diaphoresis, hyperreflexia, seizures
  - Associated with cocaine, methamphetamines, synthetic cathinones
- Alcohol or sedative/hypnotic withdrawal syndrome
  - Anxiety, shakiness, tremor, diaphoresis, vomiting, tachycardia
  - Severe withdrawal results in confusion, hallucinations, seizures
- Delirious mania
  - Neuropsychiatric syndrome of excitement, delusions, insomnia, altered level of consciousness
  - May include posturing or catatonia
  - Associated with psychotic and affective disease
- Serotonin syndrome
  - Altered mental status, neuromuscular hyperactivity, autonomic instability
  - Associated with drug-drug interactions and self-poisoning
- Neuroleptic malignant syndrome
  - Hyperthermia, increased muscle tone, diaphoresis, altered mental status, rhabdomyolysis
  - Associated with antipsychotic medication exposure, and withdrawal from dopaminergic agents
- Anticholinergic toxidrome
  - Delirium, dry mucous membranes, mydriasis, dry skin, hyperthermia
  - Follows exposure to muscarinic agents
- Heat-related illness
  - Exertional heat illness runs spectrum from heat exhaustion to heat stroke
  - Hyperthermia, delirium, rhabdomyolysis, failure of sweating mechanism (late finding)
  - Associated with exertion in high temperatures, exacerbated by mental illness and neuroleptic use
- Thyrotoxicosis
  - Heat intolerance, palpitations, anxiety, tachycardia, tremor, lid lag
  - Thyroid storm is life-threatening, causing central nervous system dysfunction, gastrointestinal-hepatic injury, and congestive heart failure

Adapted from ACEP Task Force Report on Hyperactive Delirium with Severe Agitation in Emergency Settings (2021).

2.5% to 3% of patients transported by EMS.[4,13] Among agitated patients presenting to the ED, those who have symptoms of delirium have much higher rates of clinical and adverse events, including intubation, hypotension, and need for hospital admission. The spectrum of disease in hyperactive delirium is represented in scoring systems for acute brain dysfunction. A Richmond Agitation-Sedation Scale score of +4 (combative, violent, danger to self) corresponds to patients with severe agitation, although those with lower scores may still require acute interventions to allow prehospital and hospital personnel to safely evaluate and treat.[11]

Although police use-of-force is rare, the presence of hyperactive delirium in cases that require a use-of-force intervention is disproportionately high. Depending on the specific criteria used, signs of hyperactive delirium are present in greater than 3% of use-of-force encounters, with 15% (one in six) individuals undergoing use-of-force having three or more signs at the time of the event.[3,14] Individuals with a greater number of features are less likely to have alcohol intoxication, more likely to have evidence of drug intoxication and emotional distress, and seem to be at higher risk for mortality. The mortality rate remains unknown. High estimates of mortality ranging from 8% to more than 16% are likely overestimated because of the absence of a clear definition, and publication bias in the forensic literature.[3] The actual mortality rate is probably much lower, with one retrospective study showing a significant decline in restraint-related deaths over the past several decades. The authors speculate this may be secondary to increased awareness or decreased use of prone positioning of restrained individuals, but caution that the actual death rate in restrained, severely agitated patients is so low as to limit any conclusions.[15]

PATHOPHYSIOLOGY

It is important to understand the early changes in the agitated patient that ultimately lead to agitated delirium and the far end of the spectrum resulting in death, so that effective interventions can be instituted early. The common manifestation is delirium, with multiple underlying associations: psychiatric illness, psychiatric medication withdrawal, stimulant abuse, and metabolic disorders. What ultimately leads to extremis is unknown, and likely differs between cases.[4] Most of the early literature on this syndrome came from forensic data obtained postmortem in cases attributed to hyperactive delirium. With no past or current International Classification of Diseases code, researchers often have to rely on subjective descriptors noted previously, such as severe agitation, combativeness, inappropriate nudity, and noncompliance with law enforcement. Objective clinical findings in these cases include hyperthermia, tachycardia, mydriasis, and diaphoresis. Laboratory abnormalities include hyperkalemia, acidosis, rhabdomyolysis, and acute kidney injury.[11]

More recent literature looking at the pathophysiology of hyperactive delirium hypothesizes an abnormal catecholamine response. High levels of endogenous catecholamines related to exertion and stress, combined with concomitant stimulant abuse plus physical struggle or restraint, result in hypoxia, hyperkalemia, acidosis, and autonomic dysfunction.[3,16] The common underlying pathology of the condition is dysregulation of central dopamine homeostasis.[17]

A central role of dopamine is to help continuously mediate the perceived importance of environmental events and stimuli and their internal representations. In many neuropsychiatric disorders, dopaminergic hyperactivity is linked to the symptoms of mania and psychosis. Abnormal brain activation caused by dopamine signaling is associated with cortical and subcortical hyperactivity in manic bipolar patients. Similarly, cocaine blocks the dopamine transporter protein, prolonging dopamine receptor stimulation, which leads to behavioral activation. Chronic cocaine, methamphetamine, and other psychostimulant abuse (eg, ephedrine, 3,4-methylene dioxy methamphetamine, and bath salts) results in sensitization through increased dopamine transmission and prolonged receptor stimulation.[17–20] Failure of dopamine regulation in cases of psychostimulant abuse, extreme mental stress, or an underlying psychiatric condition leads to extreme agitation, delirium, and violent behavior. Neuroanatomic links between the brain and other organ systems result in distinctive cardiorespiratory and thermal dysregulation, allowing the development of hyperthermia and cardiac dysrhythmias as a response to abnormal brain activation.[18] Other recent studies, in addition to the central dopamine hypothesis, suggest contribution of brain NADPH oxidase–derived oxidative stress in the development of cocaine-induced hyperactive delirium.[21,22]

The role of catecholamine surge resulting in hyperadrenergic state and acidosis continues to be debated. A study comparing stress biomarkers in patients with hyperactive delirium found significantly higher levels of cortisol in the severe agitation arm compared with other agitated ED patients and a control arm of volunteers exercised to exhaustion, physically restrained, and psychologically stressed by threats of application of a conducted energy weapon.[23] There were no significant differences in other stress biomarkers, such as norepinephrine, orexin (related to fight/flight response and exertional hyperthermia), dynorphin (related to stress-induced dysphoria), and copeptin (a hormonal marker of cardiovascular stress). The study itself is somewhat limited by a small sample size, and using healthy college campus volunteers in the control group, which may have contributed to the variable results in the biomarkers detected. Studies looking at markers of acidosis and catecholamine levels in simulated law enforcement encounters have shown that physical exertion tasks (sprinting, punching a heavy bag) generate greater changes in markers of acidosis and catecholamines than less lethal exposures, such as OC spray or TASER exposure.[24,25] The authors hypothesize that physical resistance when trying to control a patient with severe agitation puts them at greater risk for morbidity and mortality. Acidosis may lead to myocardial irritability and dysfunction, and catecholamine surges may lead to lethal dysrhythmia. In addition, vasodilation associated with exertion may result in decreased venous return when muscle activity ceases (ie, the patient is physically restrained). This reduces cardiac output and coronary artery perfusion at a time when elevated catecholamine levels create increased heart rate and myocardial oxygen demand. In some cases, unmasking of an unrecognized occult or partially expressed conduction abnormality, such as long QT syndrome, may result in lethal dysrhythmia and cardiovascular collapse.[26]

MANAGEMENT

Patients experiencing hyperactive delirium can go from aggressive and combative to a periarrest or perimortem state without warning. The key to effective treatment is early recognition. Given the lack of any gold standard test, physicians and other medical personnel must use their best clinical judgment when evaluating a severely agitated and delirious patient, and act expediently if indicators of hyperactive delirium are present. The differential diagnosis is broad, and without knowing the underlying cause, the critical first step in management is rapid reduction of severe agitation.[11] Although there is no strong evidence that sedation improves outcomes and lowers morbidity or mortality, diminishing the catecholamine surge and metabolic acidosis seems essential for positive short-term outcomes.[3] Be cognizant of safety concerns; patients must be prevented from injuring themselves and injuring others. Have adequate staffing at the bedside when managing severely agitated patients, to include nursing and security personnel. Physical restraints should be applied if needed. In fatal cases of hyperactive delirium, cardiac arrest often follows a struggle. Therefore, be ready to quickly supplement physical restraints with sedating medications. Supportive measures should be targeted toward specific signs and symptoms. Intravenous (IV) fluids can address dehydration from fluid loss from elevated temperature, hyperventilation, and diaphoresis. Hyperthermia, either measured or tactile, should be addressed through cool IV fluids and external cooling via ice packs or cooling blankets. Severe hyperthermia may be treated with cold water immersion, especially if exertional heat stroke is part of the differential diagnosis; however, doing so in the ED or prehospital setting may not be feasible.[27]

Three classes of medication are of use when managing ExDS: (1) benzodiazepines; (2) antipsychotics; and (3) dissociative agents, such as ketamine.[27] Benzodiazepines may be administered through the IV, intramuscular (IM), interosseous, or intranasal route and have a rapid onset, working in minutes. They bind to γ-aminobutyric acid receptors and create an inhibitory response, which is useful in patients with stimulant intoxication.[27] The primary disadvantage is respiratory depression, which may be synergistic if alcohol or other sedative medications have been ingested. The benzodiazepines studied most for the treatment of severe agitation are midazolam and lorazepam. Both show equivalent risk of oversedation or undersedation, respiratory depression, and unpredictable onset and duration of action. However, IM midazolam has a consistently faster onset of action than IM lorazepam, with a mean time to sedation of 10 to 20 minutes.[11] Respiratory monitoring with pulse oximetry and capnography should be instituted as soon as possible after administration, and the medical provider should keep a close watch on the patient's mental status and their ability to protect their airway.

Antipsychotics are used either alone or in conjunction with benzodiazepines to facilitate rapid sedation. First-generation antipsychotics, such as haloperidol and droperidol, are associated with QT prolongation, and droperidol was sidelined for years following a 2001 Food and Drug Administration Black Box Warning. However, recent studies have shown it to be safe and efficacious for treating agitated patients in the prehospital and ED settings. Doses up to 10 mg are as safe and effective as other

---

Box 2
Approach to management of hyperactive delirium with severe agitation

1. Recognize behaviors/signs of hyperactive delirium
   a. Severe psychomotor agitation
   b. Combative
   c. Failure to engage verbally/respond to verbal de-escalation
   d. Hot skin ± diaphoresis

2. Ensure staff safety
   a. Alert security
   b. Gather multiple nursing and staff personnel
   c. Use personal protective equipment (gloves, gown, mask, face shield)
   d. Have restraints and medications ready

3. Gain and maintain control of patient
   a. Physically restrain patient to facilitate immediate sedative medication administration (physical restraint is associated with sudden decompensation)
   b. Rapid sedation with intramuscular medications

4. Begin aggressive supportive care
   a. Establish intravenous or interosseous access as soon as possible
   b. Place patient on monitors (cardiac, Sao_2, $ETCO_2$)
   c. Begin fluid resuscitation
   d. Obtain core temperature (rectal or esophageal) and address hyperthermia if present with rapid cooling
   e. Closely monitor airway and hemodynamic status, with low threshold for paralysis and endotracheal intubation
   f. Address hyperdynamic state with benzodiazepines, antipsychotics, or both
   g. Place Foley catheter and monitor urine output

5. Seek out underlying causes
   a. Frequent bedside glucose monitoring
   b. Obtain electrocardiogram, chest radiograph; consider neuroimaging (computed tomography), especially if focal neurodeficits are present
   c. Serum studies to include complete blood count, electrolytes, renal function, liver function, coagulation studies, creatine kinase, troponin, ethanol
   d. Send urine for dipstick and microscopic
   e. Qualitative urine toxicology screen of low utility, but may be a useful screen for sympathomimetic abuse
   f. Hospitalize in intensive care unit or step-down unit

Table 1
Medications for initial sedation in hyperactive delirium

- Optimal strategy is immediate IM administration.
- Goal is rapid sedation.
- Consider reduced dosing for IV/interosseous administration, acknowledging risk of inadequate sedation.
- Sedation should be followed by aggressive airway and hemodynamic support.

Medication	Dose	Onset (Approximate)	Pros	Cons
Midazolam (Versed)	5–10 mg	3 min IV, 10–20 min IM	More rapid onset than lorazepam	Respiratory depression
Droperidol (Inapsine)	5–10 mg	3–10 min IV, 10–20 min IM	Rapid onset, less respiratory depression than midazolam	QTc prolongation (rare, little evidence for harm)
Olanzapine (Zyprexa)	5–10 mg	5–10 min IV, 10–20 min IM	Rapid onset, less respiratory depression than benzodiazepines	Less well-studied than other agents
Ketamine	2 mg/kg IV, 4–5 mg/kg IM	30 s IV, 2–15 min IM	Fastest time to sedation	Greater risk of respiratory adverse events than droperidol or olanzapine

Abbreviations: IM, intramuscular; IV, intravenous.

medications. When doses greater than 2.5 mg are used, cardiac monitoring should be instituted as soon as feasible.[28,29] Olanzapine in doses up to 10 mg IM is also an excellent option, with equivalent or superior control of agitation than haloperidol. Both droperidol and olanzapine provide more rapid sedation than haloperidol, with a mean time to sedation ranging from 10 to 22 minutes, making them the current first-line antipsychotic medications for severe agitation.[11]

Ketamine is a dissociative anesthetic that prevents the higher brain centers from perceiving visual, auditory, or painful stimuli. Onset is rapid, and it may be delivered intravenously or intramuscularly. When administered intramuscularly, onset of action is about 5 minutes, making it ideal for gaining control of severely agitated patients in the field and in the ED. Side effects include hypersalivation, nausea, emergence reactions (which is countered with benzodiazepines), and rarely, laryngospasm.[30–32] Obviously, these patients may be critically ill and are at risk for rapid deterioration, warranting hospitalization and ongoing observation and treatment, initially in the intensive care setting.

Following several high-profile cases of individuals who died after prehospital treatment with ketamine, there have been calls to limit its use. Along with these anecdotal incidents, there has been concern for excessive airway loss and need for intubation when severely agitated patients are treated with ketamine by EMS. However, literature showing harm is actually rare, with a single case of successfully managed laryngospasm being cited, and intubation being performed secondary to subjective criteria.[33] The need for intubation seems to be highest in patients with sympathomimetic ingestion, and also associated with higher doses of ketamine.[34,35] A recent study looked at safety of ketamine at subdissociative doses for pain control and dissociative doses for severe agitation/delirium, accounting for such issues as concomitant medication use and patient comorbidities. They found ketamine had an excellent safety profile, with few neuropsychiatric adverse events and low rates of endotracheal intubation.[36] Findings in a meta-analysis looking at the safest and most effective means of rapid tranquilization of agitated ED patients suggest that ketamine is the superior agent to droperidol.[37] Given its rapid onset and safety profile, ketamine should be considered a first-line medication for hyperactive delirium. Prehospital providers and physicians should be ready to manage any potential airway problems that may arise secondary to pharmacologic sedation, coingestions, or the underlying hemodynamic lability associated with hyperactive delirium (**Box 2**, **Table 1**).

CLINICS CARE POINTS

- Safety of the patient and of the medical providers is paramount in presentations of hyperactive delirium with severe agitation, and the ED should be prepared to manage these patients with adequate staffing, restraints, and pharmacologic sedatives.

- The emergency physician must institute cardiac and respiratory monitoring and anticipate rapid vascular collapse and airway loss in patients with severe agitation, especially after sedative medications are administered.

- Treatment should focus on rapid sedation, followed by airway protection, supportive measures, and cooling of hyperthermic patients.

- Ketamine's rapid onset of action, efficacy in reducing severe agitation, and safety profile make it the ideal first-line medication for hyperactive delirium in the prehospital or ED setting, although droperidol or midazolam are also reasonable choices.

DISCLOSURE

The author has nothing to disclose.

REFERENCES

1. Samuel E, Williams RB, Ferrell RB. Excited delirium: consideration of selected medical and psychiatric issues. Neuropsychiatric Dis Treat 2009;5:61.
2. Takeuchi A, Ahern TL, Henderson SO. Excited delirium. West J Emerg Med 2011; 12(1):77.
3. Gonin P, Beysard N, Yersin B, et al. Excited delirium: a systematic review. Acad Emerg Med 2018;25(5):552–65.
4. Vilke GM, DeBard ML, Chan TC, et al. Excited delirium syndrome (ExDS): defining based on a review of the literature. J Emerg Med 2012;43(5):897–905.
5. Byard RW. Ongoing issues with the diagnosis of excited delirium. Forensic Sci Med Pathol 2018;14:149–215.
6. ACEP Excited Delirium Task Force (2009). White paper report on excited delirium syndrome. American College of Emergency Physicians. Available at: https://www.acep.org/administration/ems-resources/. Accessed August 1, 2022.
7. New AMA policy opposes "excited delirium" diagnosis." Available at: https://www.ama-assn.org/press-center/press-releases/new-ama-policy-opposes-excited-delirium-diagnosis. Accessed August 1, 2022.
8. Applebaum P. Excited delirium, ketamine, and deaths in police custody. Psychiatr Serv 2022;73(7):827–9.
9. Fiscella K, Pinals D, Shields C. "Excited delirium," erroneous concepts, dehumanizing language, false narratives, and threat to Black lives. Acad Emerg Med 2022; 29(7):911–3.
10. Saadi A, Naples-Mitchell J, Batia B, et al. End the use of "excited delirium" as a cause of death in police custody, Lancet, 399 (10329), 2022, 1028–1030.
11. ACEP Task Force Report on Hyperactive Delirium with Severe Agitation in Emergency Settings (2021). American College of Emergency Physicians. Available at: https://www.acep.org/by-medical-focus/hyperactive-delirium/. Accessed August 1, 2022.
12. Baldwin S, Hall C, Bennell C, et al. Distinguishing features of excited delirium syndrome in non-fatal use of force encounters. Journal of Forensic and Legal Medicine 2016;41:21–7.
13. Miner JR, Klein LR, Cole JB, et al. The characteristics and prevalence of agitation in an urban county emergency department. Ann Emerg Med 2018;72(4):361–70.
14. Hall CA, Kader AS, McHale AMD, et al. Frequency of signs of excited delirium syndrome in subjects undergoing police use of force: descriptive evaluation of a prospective, consecutive cohort. Journal of Forensic and Legal Medicine 2013;20(2):102–7.
15. Michaud A. Restraint related deaths and excited delirium syndrome in Ontario (2004–2011). Journal of Forensic and Legal Medicine 2016;41:30–5.
16. Strote J, Walsh M, Auerbach D, et al. Medical conditions and restraint in patients experiencing excited delirium. AJEM (Am J Emerg Med) 2014;32(9):1093–6.
17. Mash DC. Excited delirium and sudden death: a syndromal disorder at the extreme end of the neuropsychiatric continuum. Front Physiol 2016;7:435.
18. Mash DC, Duque L, Pablo J, et al. Brain biomarkers for identifying excited delirium as a cause of sudden death. Forensic Sci Int 2009;190(1–3):e13–9.
19. Penders TM. The syndrome of excited delirium following use of "bath salts". J Clin Psychiatry 2013;74(5):518.

20. Penders TM, Gestring RE, Vilensky DA. Excited delirium following use of synthetic cathinones (bath salts). Gen Hosp Psychiatr 2012;34(6):647–50.

21. Turillazzi E. Involvement of the NADPH oxidase NOX2–derived brain oxidative stress in an unusual fatal case of cocaine-related neurotoxicity associated with excited delirium syndrome. J Clin Psychopharmacol 2016;36(5):513–7.

22. Schiavone S, Neri M, Mhillaj E, et al. The role of the NADPH oxidase derived brain oxidative stress in the cocaine-related death associated with excited delirium: a literature review. Toxicology letters 2016;258:29–35.

23. Vilke GM, Mash DC, Pardo M, et al. EXCITATION study: unexplained in-custody deaths: evaluating biomarkers of stress and agitation. Journal of forensic and legal medicine 2019;66:100–6.

24. Ho JD, Dawes DM, Nelson RS, et al. Acidosis and catecholamine evaluation following simulated law enforcement "use of force" encounters. Acad Emerg Med 2010;17(7):e60–8.

25. Ho JD, Dawes DM, Nystrom PC, et al. Markers of acidosis and stress in a sprint versus a conducted electrical weapon. Forensic Sci Int 2013;l233(1–3):84–9.

26. Bozeman WP, Ali K, Winslow JE. Long QT syndrome unmasked in an adult subject presenting with excited delirium. The Journal of emergency medicine 2013; 44(2):e207–10.

27. Vilke GM, Bozeman WP, Dawes DM, et al. Excited delirium syndrome (ExDS): treatment options and considerations. Journal of Forensic and Legal Medicine 2012;19(3):117–21.

28. Macht M, Mull AC, McVaney KE, et al. Comparison of droperidol and haloperidol for use by paramedics: assessment of safety and effectiveness. Prehosp Emerg Care 2014;18(3):375–80.

29. Perkins J, Ho J. Safety of droperidol use in the emergency department: clinical practice statement. American Academy of Emergency Medicine 2013;9(7).

30. Riddell J, Tran A, Bengiamin R, et al. Ketamine as a first-line treatment for severely agitated emergency department patients. Am J Emerg Med 2017; 35(7):1000–4.

31. Ho JD, Smith SW, Nystrom PC, et al. Successful management of excited delirium syndrome with prehospital ketamine: two case examples. Prehosp Emerg Care 2013;17(2):274–9.

32. Scheppke KA, Braghiroli J, Shalaby M, et al. Prehospital use of IM ketamine for sedation of violent and agitated patients. West J Emerg Med 2014;15(7):736.

33. Kitch B. Out-of-hospital ketamine: review of a growing trend in patient care. J Am Coll Emerg Physicians Open 2020;1(3):183–9.

34. Kim H, Leonard J, Corwell B, et al. Safety and efficacy of pharmacologic agents used for rapid tranquilization of emergency department patients with acute agitation or excited delirium, Expert Opin Drug Saf, 20 (2), 2021, 123–138.

35. Solano J, Clayton L, Parks D, et al. Prehospital ketamine administration for excited delirium with illicit substance co-ingestion and subsequent intubation in the emergency department, Prehosp Disaster Med, 36 (6), 2021, 697–701.

36. Mo H, Campbell M, Fertel B, et al. Ketamine safety and use in the emergency department for pain and agitation/delirium: a health system experience, West J Emerg Med, 21 (2), 2020, 272–281.

37. deSouza I, Thode Jr H, Shrestha P, et al. Rapid tranquilization of the agitated patient in the emergency department: a systematic review and network meta-analysis, Am J Emerg Med, 51, 2022, 363–373.

Substance Use Disorder

Kaitlyn R. Swimmer, MD[a], Stephen Sandelich, MD[a,b],*

KEYWORDS

- Substance use disorder • Alcohol • Opiate • Medicated-assisted treatment

KEY POINTS

- Substance use disorder (SUD) is widespread, posing serious health risks, with alcohol use disorder being the most prevalent type worldwide.
- Alcohol withdrawal in adolescents and adults is treated with benzodiazepines, while opioid withdrawal can be managed with buprenorphine.
- Medication-assisted treatments, complemented by multimodal therapies, demonstrate effectiveness in SUD management for both adults and adolescents.
- Treatment strategies for alcohol and opioid use disorders vary by age group, involving specific medications and therapy components to tackle their severity levels.
- The prevalence of polysubstance use necessitates holistic assessment of substance use, and legal protections exist to ensure patient confidentiality regarding SUD disclosures.

INTRODUCTION

Substance use disorders (SUDs) are a prevalent category of disorders that carry major stigma both in the general population and within the medical community.[1] They are associated with significant morbidity and mortality. According to the National Survey on Drug Use and Health (NSDUH), among people aged 12 years and older, 58.7% have used tobacco, alcohol, or an illicit drug in the past month.[2] In this group, 22.2% reported that they were binge alcohol users in the past month, with these numbers being higher (31.4%) in young adults from ages 18 to 25 years; 21.4% of respondents reported that they have used illicit drugs in the past year, with marijuana being the most common. In 2020, about 40.3 million people reported a diagnosis of an SUD based on the Diagnostic and Statistical Manual of Mental Disorders-5 (DSM-5) criteria.

There is a significant overlap with SUD and many mental health conditions such as post-traumatic stress disorder (PTSD), personality disorders, depression, anxiety,

[a] Department of Pediatrics, Penn State Health Milton S. Hershey Medical Center, 500 University Drive, Hershey, PA 17033, USA; [b] Emergency Medicine, Penn State Health Milton S. Hershey Medical Center, 500 University Drive, Hershey, PA 17033, USA
* Corresponding author. Penn State Health Milton S. Hershey Medical Center, 500 University Drive, Hershey, PA 17033.
E-mail address: ssandelich@pennstatehealth.psu.edu

Emerg Med Clin N Am 42 (2024) 53–67
https://doi.org/10.1016/j.emc.2023.06.023
0733-8627/24/© 2023 Elsevier Inc. All rights reserved.

emed.theclinics.com

schizophrenia, and psychosis.[3-6] Many patients with SUD and coexisting mental health conditions use emergency department services frequently, as they experience multiple barriers to health care. The emergency department is used as a medical home for many patients, with reports of up to half of all emergency department visits relating to substance use/abuse.[7,8]

There has been an increase in the amount of substance use and abuse both in the general as well as the adolescent population with the COVID pandemic.[9,10] Many patients report that their substance use has increased as a coping mechanism secondary to anxiety related to the pandemic. There has also been an increase in the number of patients reporting regular alcohol use ranging from 21.7% to 72.9%.[11] Adolescents were particularly susceptible to stressors brought on by the COVID pandemic.[12-16] Adolescent-specific risk factors include stay-at-home schooling and disturbances from day-to-day life. The full impact on adolescents with regard to substance use/abuse is still not completely known.

Clinical Assessment

The emergency department is often the first and sometimes only point of access many patients have with the health care system. Given this limitation, various screening tools have been implemented in the emergency department to identify patients at risk for SUD as strategies for intervention.[17,18] The American College of Emergency Physicians has published a policy statement stating that "ACEP believes emergency medical professionals are positioned and qualified to mitigate the consequences of alcohol abuse through screening programs, brief intervention, and referral to treatment."[19] Brief screening questionnaires have been developed in order to help the emergency medicine physician screen for both alcohol and other substances. Validated alcohol screening include the Alcohol Use Disorders Identification Test,[20,21] the CAGE,[22,23] and the single-question National Institute on Alcohol Abuse and Alcoholism test.[24] There tests are less validated screening tools for illicit substances; however, a single question regarding illicit drug use has been evaluated in the primary care setting (How many times in the past year have you used an illegal drug or used a prescription medication for nonmedical reasons?) and may be a viable screen in the emergency department. This single question was reported to have a sensitivity of 100% and a specificity of 73.5% for detecting an SUD.[25]

Positive screens should prompt a more extensive assessment for SUD. A full substance use history involves discussing which substances are being used, the amount, and frequency. Prior diagnoses and treatment of SUDs should also be determined. When possible, obtaining corroborating information from outside sources such as the patient's family members and prior medical records can be beneficial.

In determining the severity of a patient's SUD, the clinician needs to establish which substances are being used. Many patients endorse polysubstance drug use, and SUD of one substance increases risk for concurrent substances being used, and in fact many patients endorse polysubstance use when asked.[26-29] In 2019 nearly half of drug overdose deaths involved multiple drugs, with the most common combination being opioids and stimulants.[30] To gain a full understanding of the types of substances a person may be abusing, the physician should assess for a wide range of substances including caffeine, tobacco/nicotine, alcohol, prescription pain medications, marijuana, and finally illicit drugs including cocaine, opioids, hallucinogens, and inhalants. For each substance that the patient endorses using, it is important to ask about the use pattern including last use, frequency, and estimated amount. In addition to the types of substances being used, the route of administration including oral, smoking, intranasal, subcutaneous, intramuscular, and intravenous should be obtained.

There is a strong association between mental health disorders and substance use.[31–33] Patients may present with a range of comorbid diagnoses including depression, bipolar, anxiety, PTSD, schizophrenia, and/or attention-deficit hyperactivity disorder. Patients actively experiencing withdrawal symptoms may present with signs or symptoms similar to anxiety, including agitation, behavioral changes, inability to sleep, and hemodynamic lability. Each specific drug has a specific time period of withdrawal symptoms and a specific withdrawal toxidrome.

A SUD can alter multiple body systems and functions. Patients may develop comorbid medical conditions based on the substances or the route of administration. During the general assessment and evaluation, the clinician should be alert to signs of past drug use including scars and injection sites, atrophy of the nasal mucosa, and evidence of acute intoxication and/or withdrawal. There are many medical conditions that may arise from substance use and abuse as outlined in **Table 1**. A full understanding of a patient's medical history is imperative to develop a complete treatment plan for their SUD.

Laboratory assessment of a patient for substance use in the emergency department for SUD is complicated. Testing a patient's urine and blood for specific substances in the emergency department is often practiced; however, this rarely changes management. A urine drug immunoassay may reveal recent drug use but has low specificity and sensitivity and does not give detail regarding the amount and pattern of substance use.[34] Even when patients are able and willing to communicate their use patterns, there is a wide variation between self-reported amount of substances ingested compared with drug screen results.[35–40] Every substance has a range of days during which it may continue to test positive in a urine drug assay as noted in **Table 2**.[41,42] Most urine commercial drug screens are immunoassays that are simple to use, quick, and relatively cheap. Although they may lead to a true positive in cases of substances being present in the urine, many classes of commonly used medications may lead to a false-positive result in most common urine drug immunoassays.[43] Examples of classes of drugs leading to false positives include antihistamines, antidepressants, antibiotics, analgesics, antipsychotics, and nonprescription agents.[44] All positive results on a urine drug immunoassay should have confirmatory testing in the form of chromatography/mass spectrometry. These secondary tests may be reflexively run through the laboratory or many need to be ordered by the clinician. A further drawback to the standard urine drug screen is that many synthetic or designer drugs are not identified on the screen. Substances that are not commonly detected on most urine drug screens include nonbenzodiazepine hypnotics, ketamine, mescaline, psilocybin, gamma-hydroxybutyrate, synthetic cannabinoids, tryptamines, phenethylamine derivatives (bath salts), and imidazoline receptor agonists (clonidine). For example, marijuana is typically detected in the urine on most standard assays, although most synthetic cannabinoids are not able to be detected.[45,46] If concerns about a specific substance persist after initial evaluation, the urine drug screen is often not sufficient to rule in or out substance use.[47,48]

Legal Issues Pertaining to Drug Testing

Substance use evaluations are often fraught with stigma both at personal and the societal levels. Patients may not want to disclose their substance use history or may significantly minimize it. Given the nature of these evaluations, there must be a balance between the physician's respect for patient autonomy and duty to care for the patient. In general, physicians do not ask a patient's permission for every individual test. However, urine drug screening should be viewed somewhat differently. Patients may be

Table 1 General medical conditions resulting from substance use and abuse	
Cardiovascular	Hypertension
	Cardiomyopathy
	Endocarditis
	Heart failure
Gastrointestinal/Renal	Pancreatitis
	Cirrhosis
	Chronic liver failure
	Kidney failure
	Hepatitis B
	Hepatitis C
Central Nervous System	Dementia
	Memory and attention impairments
	Intracranial hemorrhage
	Cerebral vasculitis
	Ischemic events
	Stroke
	Traumatic brain injury
Pulmonary	Bronchospasm
	Chronic obstructive lung disease
	Pulmonary edema
	Pneumonia
	Hypersensitivity pneumonitis
	Barotrauma
	Hemoptysis
	Tuberculosis
Hematologic	Anemia
	Bone marrow dysfunction
Sexually Transmitted Infection	HIV
	Syphilis
	Gonorrhea
	Genital warts

Abbreviation: HIV, human immunodeficiency virus.

concerned about their employer or insurer discovering their results. Given the sensitive nature of drug testing, it is best practice to obtain informed consent before obtaining drug testing specifically when assessing for SUDs; however, this is often not done in clinical practice. In response to these privacy concerns the federal government passed legislation, and the Department of Health and Human services issued a set of regulations to protect patients' information regarding substance abuse. These regulations severely limit the type of information that can be disclosed regarding disclosure of substance abuse and their treatment.

Case law can bring to light some pitfalls. In *Ballensky v. Flattum-Riemers*[49] the police were provided positive drug results from a patient without express consent. The physician noted that the patient was not clinically intoxicated, and the court upheld that the patient could sue the physician for a breach of confidentiality. Obtaining and documenting informed consent in cases relating to drug testing is of paramount importance. When patients refuse treatment even if mandated by their employer or law enforcement, physicians should abide by their wishes. The case of *Sharp v Cleveland Clinic* brings this to light. In this case an on-duty nurse was asked to provide a urine sample after being suspected of being intoxicated. She subsequently sued the

Table 2
Timing window for specific substances in common urine drug immunoassays (days)

Amphetamines	Methamphetamine	3
	Amphetamine	3
	MDMA	2
	Pseudoephedrine	5
Barbiturates	Phenobarbital	15
	Butalbital	7
	Pentobarbital	3
Benzodiazepines	Diazepam	10
	Alprazolam	5
	Lorazepam	5
	Clonazepam	5
	Midazolam	2
Cocaine	—	<12H
LSD	Lysergic diethylamide	<1H
	2-Oxo-3-hydroxy-LSD	5
Opioids (Natural)	Heroin	3
	Morphine	3
	Codeine	3
Opioids (Semisynthetic)	Hydrocodone	3
	Hydromorphone	3
	Oxycodone	3
	Oxymorphone	3
Opioids (Synthetic)	Fentanyl	3
	Methadone	7
	Buprenorphine	7
Phencyclidine	—	8
THC	—	3–30

Abbreviations: LSD, lysergic acid diethylamide; THC, tetrahydrocannabinol.

hospital for false imprisonment; however, the claim was denied because informed consent was documented, and the patient was free to leave at any time. Once testing has been obtained, patient confidentiality always must remain a priority. The default response for a request for results must be only with express patient agreement unless presented with a warrant from law enforcement. If concerns arise, it is suggested to seek advice from hospital legal counsel.

Family history and social history also play a significant role in evaluating the emergency patient for SUD. Unfortunately, patients who are experiencing substance use issues often have significant social risk factors, and identifying these factors can lead to efforts for treating SUD and mitigating its negative effects. A thorough family and social history can uncover many of these risks and can evaluate what protective factors the patient is experiencing. Risk factors are characterized as biological, psychological, family, community, or cultural factors that are associated with higher likelihood of negative outcomes. Both risk and protective factors can be found in relationship, community, and societal contexts. Individual factors include family history of SUD, child abuse, and maltreatment and life partners and peers with SUD. Community factors include living in neighborhoods with high levels of poverty and violence and where there is a high availability of drugs and alcohol. A major risk factor for the development of SUD is a family history of SUD with increased rates up to 75%.[50–53]

Adverse childhood experiences (ACE) have been shown to be correlated with higher levels of substance use and SUD although the exact mechanism is not completely elucidated.[54,55] ACE are traumatic childhood events that have negative long-term effects on health and well-being. Adverse childhood experiences can be categorized into abuse, household challenges, and neglect. Abuse includes emotional, physical, and sexual abuse. Household challenges include substance abuse in the household, mental illness in the household, parental separation, incarcerated household member, and domestic violence. Neglect includes both emotional and physical neglect. It has been shown that there is a correlation with the number of ACE that a patient reports and many leading causes of morbidity and mortality as adults, including many cancers, ischemic heart disease, and stroke.[56,57] Increasing ACE levels are also highly associated with both lifetime development and early adoption of illicit substance use. In a study of primary care patients self-reporting their ACE, each ACE reported increased the likelihood of early initiation of drug use by 2- to 4-fold, and a higher ACE score was correlated with higher lifetime SUD rates.

Diagnosis

A diagnosis of SUD is based on the patient meeting the diagnostic criteria defined by the DSM-5.[58,59] The criteria for the DSM-5 diagnosis for SUD are listed in **Box 1** and are broken down into impaired control over substance use (1–4), social impairment (5–7), risky use (8–9), and pharmacologic criteria (10–11). A patient may be diagnosed with an SUD for multiple drugs. The substances that are recognized by the DSM-5 as potential drugs of abuse include alcohol, caffeine, cannabis, hallucinogens, inhalants, opioids, sedative, hypnotics, stimulants, and tobacco. The DSM-5 specifies severity modifiers including mild, moderate, and severe. Mild SUD involved 2 to 3 criteria, moderate includes 4 to 5 criteria, and severe includes 6 or more.

Approach for Treatment of Specific Substance Use Disorder—Alcohol Use Disorder

Alcohol use disorder (AUD) is the most common SUD with an estimated worldwide prevalence of 100 million people worldwide. AUD is unfortunately severely undertreated, with only about 7% of adults receiving appropriate pharmacotherapy and or psychotherapy treatments.[60,61] Patients with a mild AUD may receive benefit from monotherapy and from psychosocial interventions such as brief motivational counseling and mutual help groups. In patients with moderate or severe disorders, concurrent pharmacologic treatments are often required, and even with a mix of therapies, up to 70% of patients will return to alcohol use. There are currently only 3 pharmacologic treatments that are approved by the US Food and Drug Administration for AUD treatment, including acamprosate, naltrexone, and disulfiram.

When initiating treatment of patients with moderate-to-severe AUD, naltrexone is generally the drug of choice. Naltrexone is a mu opioid receptor antagonist. Through attenuation of the alcohol-induced dopaminergic system, naltrexone can modulate the rewarding effects of alcohol, leading to a reduced alcohol consumption.[62,63] Naltrexone is preferred as a first-line agent because it can be dosed on a daily dosing schedule, and treatment can be initiated while the patient is still drinking. There have been multiple studies showing that a combination of psychotherapy and naltrexone as well as monotherapy with naltrexone can reduce alcohol consumption in patients with AUD.[64–71] In patients who experience significant side effects from naltrexone or have difficulty with adherence to daily medications, extended-release naltrexone is an option. This formulation is administered once monthly by a medical professional and does have some data showing reduced alcohol use.[72,73]

Box 1
Criteria for diagnosing and classifying substance use disorders

1. Consuming the substance in larger amounts and for a longer amount of time than intended.

2. Persistent desire to cut down or regulate use. The individual may have unsuccessfully attempted to stop in the past.

3. Spending a great deal of time obtaining, using, or recovering from the effects of substance use.

4. Experiencing craving, a pressing desire to use the substance.

5. Substance use impairs ability to fulfill major obligations at work, school, or home.

6. Continued use of the substance despite it causing significant social or interpersonal problems.

7. Reduction or discontinuation of recreational, social, or occupational activities because of substance use.

8. Recurrent substance use in physically unsafe environments.

9. Persistent substance use despite knowledge that it may cause or exacerbate physical or psychological problems.

10. *Tolerance*: individual requires increasingly higher doses of the substance to achieve the desired effect, or the usual dose has a reduced effect; individuals may build tolerance to specific symptoms at different rates.

11. *Withdrawal*: a collection of signs and symptoms that occurs when blood and tissue levels of the substance decrease. Individuals are likely to seek the substance to relieve symptoms. No documented withdrawal symptoms from hallucinogens, phencyclidine, or inhalants.

In patients with a contraindication to naltrexone, acamprosate is a reasonable treatment option. The specific mechanism of action is not fully clear; however, it is thought it acts on the glutamatergic system as an N-methyl-D-aspartate receptor partial co-agonist.[74–76] There are mixed data on the efficacy of acamprosate in the treatment of AUD, with some studies showing a reduction in rates of alcohol consumption, whereas others showing no difference compared with a placebo.[71,77–79]

Disulfiram was the first medication approved for AUD and works through inhibiting aldehyde dehydrogenase. When alcohol is taken in the presence of disulfiram, an adverse reaction characterized by nausea, vomiting, sweating, flushing, and heart palpitation occurs. Given the unpleasant nature of these symptoms, disulfiram has a relatively poor adherence rate and is often not recommended for a first-line treatment of AUD.[80,81]

Alcohol withdrawal syndrome is a potentially lethal complication of abrupt reduction/cessation in alcohol usage in someone with AUD. The prevalence of AUD is astounding, as it is the seventh highest cause of morbidity and mortality in the world.[82] To put this in perspective, between 2% and 7% of patients with AUD who are hospitalized will develop alcohol withdrawal syndrome severe enough to require pharmacologic management. The more severe the underlying AUD and the longer the patient goes without alcohol or medical management, the more likely they are to have severe alcohol withdrawal.

The DSM-5 defines the diagnostic criteria for alcohol withdrawal as 2 or more defining symptoms/signs that develop within a few hours to days after cessation of or reduction in alcohol use that has been heavy and prolonged.[59] These signs/symptoms include autonomic hyperactivity, increased hand tremor, insomnia, nausea/

vomiting, transient visual/tactile/auditory hallucinations, psychomotor agitation, anxiety, and generalized tonic-clonic seizures. Alcohol withdrawal is classified into 3 main categories: mild, moderate, and severe. Mild withdrawal generally present within a few hours of the last alcoholic drink and resolves within 24 to 48 hours. Mild withdrawal may be managed conservatively without benzodiazepines or barbiturates. Moderate alcohol withdrawal, also known as alcohol hallucinosis, typically present within 12 to 24 hours after the last drink and resolves in another 24 to 48 hours. Severe withdrawal includes both withdrawal seizures and withdrawal delirium (delirium tremens). It is critically important to treat withdrawal, as progression to Delirium Tremens is associated with a mortality rate of 1% to 4%.[82,83]

Benzodiazepines continue to be first-line treatment of alcohol withdrawal with moderate-to-severe symptoms.[83] Consideration must be given, as they have a relatively short half-life and high potential for misuse.[82] No particular benzodiazepines are recommended; however, longer-acting agents are generally preferred. If a patient will be discharged on benzodiazepines, both the patient and their caregiver must be educated on potential risks, including the dangers of drug-drug interactions between benzodiazepines and other central nervous system depressants, the risk of combining benzodiazepines and alcohol, and the risks of driving/using heavy machinery while under the influence of benzodiazepines. Alternate medications for moderate alcohol withdrawal include carbamazepine or gabapentin. Phenobarbital is an appropriate alternative for severe withdrawal.

When possible and not limited by the cognition of the patient, treatment of both the underlying SUD and the acute withdrawal should be taken together with appropriate pharmacological treatments offered for AUD.

Approach for Treatment of Specific Substance Use Disorder—Opiate Use Disorder

The DSM-5 defines opioid withdrawal syndrome as 3 or more defining symptoms/signs that cause clinically significant distress or impairment in social/occupational/other important areas of functioning and that develop within a few minutes to days after the cessation of/reduction in opioid use that has been heavy and prolonged OR the administration of an opioid antagonist after a period of opioid use. These signs/symptoms include dysphoric mood, lacrimation/rhinorrhea, piloerection/pupillary dilation/sweating, myalgia, diarrhea, nausea/vomiting, insomnia, autonomic hyperactivity (tachypnea, hyperreflexia, tachycardia, sweating, hypertension, hyperthermia), and yawning.

Treatment of opiate use disorder consists of a combination of pharmacotherapy and psychosocial treatment. This treatment generally requires long-term follow-up to ensure adequate results, with some treatment protocols lasting between 6 and 12 months. In addition to treating the opiate withdrawal symptoms and the underlying opioid use disorder, all patients who are being treated or evaluated for opioid use disorder should also be provided home naloxone in case of accidental overdose. The opiate withdrawal syndrome is a potentially lethal complication due to abrupt reduction/cessation in opioid usage in someone with opioid use disorder.[84,85] Unlike alcohol withdrawal, opioid withdrawal, although potentially very unpleasant, is rarely life-threatening. Opioid withdrawal syndrome is also broken down into categories based on severity: mild, moderate, moderately severe, and severe.

Current clinical practice guidelines recommend that gold-standard and first-line pharmacotherapy for opioid withdrawal syndrome is buprenorphine. Other medications including clonidine, methadone, and naltrexone are options; however, they have been shown to have either less efficacy or worse safety profile. Buprenorphine can be safely initiated in the emergency department and should be considered, as studies have shown improved outcomes in patients with opioid withdrawal syndrome who were initiated on buprenorphine in the emergency department.[86] Buprenorphine is a partial opiate agonist with high affinity for mu receptors. When it activates the mu receptors it will provide an adequate opioid effect while having a very low risk of respiratory depression and giving less of the euphoric effects as traditional opiates. Naloxone is often formulated with buprenorphine in order to act as an abuse deterrent. Buprenorphine therapy for opiate withdrawal can be initiated in the emergency department; however, care must be taken in patients who have recently taken other opiates, specifically long-acting opiates such as methadone. Buprenorphine can displace other opiates at the mu receptor and precipitate withdrawal. With this limitation in mind, both a combination of a scoring of a patient's withdrawal as well as a history of their last opiate use must be used to determine when it is safe to initiate buprenorphine therapy. Treatment doses with buprenorphine typically begin between 4 and 8 mg given in a sublingual film; however, it can be increased up to 24 mg to control cravings. Once buprenorphine therapy has been initiated, the patient's care must be handed off to a provider comfortable in the long-term care of patients with SUD. Most patients on buprenorphine therapy will maintain for months until they can be weaned off, and unfortunately, relapses are a common occurrence.[87]

Substance Use Disorder in the Adolescent Population

Although SUDs ore often thought of in relation to the adult populations, they also have a significant prevalence in adolescents. SUD in adolescents can have long-lasting ramifications. Identifying and intervening in this group is particularly important. According to the 2019 NSDUH report, more than 15,000,000 adolescents (roughly 40% of the adolescent population) aged 12 to 20 years reported that they had used alcohol at some point in their life, and more than 12,000,000 (roughly 32% of adolescent population) reported illicit drug use at some point in their life.[88] According to the same report, in 2020 alone about 3,780,000 adolescents (about 10% of adolescent population) aged 12 to 20 years were diagnosed with SUD, about 75% of whom were classified as needing treatment of their SUD.[88]

Treatment strategies for adolescents with withdrawal and/or SUD are not well researched or tested, so typically the adult protocols are used in this population. The signs and symptoms of withdrawal are similar for adolescents and adults. As in adults, first-line treatment of alcohol withdrawal in adolescents is benzodiazepines along with other supportive care.[89] Current pharmacotherapy recommendations based on limited clinical trial data for adolescents withdrawing from opioids is buprenorphine, same as in adults.[90]

As with adult treatment strategies, it is important to treat the underlying SUDs in adolescents. Unfortunately, research and supportive data are lacking with regard to maintenance treatments of SUDs in adolescents. Based on anecdotal evidence and efficacy data extrapolated from research on maintenance treatment of adults with SUD, both pharmacotherapy and psychosocial treatment is recommended for SUD in adolescents.[89,91] If opioid use disorder is mild, adolescents seem to benefit from treatment with naltrexone in addition to counseling/therapy, although there are no clinical trials to support the efficacy of naltrexone as a treatment of SUD in adolescents.[91] If opioid use disorder is moderate/severe, adolescents have been shown in clinical trials to benefit from buprenorphine in addition to psychosocial treatment.[90] Unlike adults, however, other medications such as clonidine and methadone are not recommended, as they have not been found in limited trials to be effective.[90,91] There is extremely limited data regarding maintenance treatment of AUD in adolescents, but some limited emerging data have shown brief interventions to have some efficacy.[89]

CLINICS CARE POINTS

- SUDs are a very common disorder in emergency department patients.
- Consider screening for SUD in all patients being evaluated in the emergency department.
- The emergency department is an appropriate venue to initiate treatment of both alcohol and opiate use disorders.
- Buprenorphine is the first-line therapy for opiate withdrawal and can be safely initiated in the emergency department.

DISCLOSURE

The authors have nothing to disclose.

REFERENCES

1. Ahern J, Stuber J, Galea S. Stigma, discrimination and the health of illicit drug users. Drug Alcohol Depend 2007;88(2–3):188–96.
2. Park-Lee REA. Key Substance Use and Mental Health Indicators in the United States: Results from the 2020 National Survey on Drug Use and Health. HHS Publication No PEP19-5068, NSDUH Series H-54. 2019;170:51-58. Available at: https://www.samhsa.gov/data/. Accessed November 29, 2022.
3. Martínez-Raga J, Didia-Attas J, Ruiz M, et al. Post-traumatic stress disorder and substance use disorder: epidemiology, nature and neurobiology. Vertex 2005; 16(63):325–31.
4. Donald F, Arunogiri S, Lubman DI. Substance use and borderline personality disorder: fostering hope in the face of complexity. Australas Psychiatr 2019;27(6): 569–72.
5. Regnart J, Truter I, Meyer A. Critical exploration of co-occurring Attention-Deficit/ Hyperactivity Disorder, mood disorder and Substance Use Disorder. Expert Rev Pharmacoecon Outcomes Res 2017;17(3):275–82.
6. Wisdom JP, Manuel JI, Drake RE. Substance Use Disorder Among People With First-Episode Psychosis: A Systematic Review of Course and Treatment. Psychiatr Serv 2011;62(9). https://doi.org/10.1176/appi.ps.62.9.1007.
7. Crane EH. Highlights of the 2011 Drug Abuse Warning Network (DAWN) Findings on Drug-Related Emergency Department Visits.; 2013. Available at: https://www.samhsa.gov/data/sites/default/files/DAWN096/DAWN096/SR096EDHighlights 2010.htm. Accessed November 29, 2022.
8. Zhang X, Wang N, Hou F, et al. Emergency department visits by patients with substance use disorder in the United States. West J Emerg Med 2021;22(5):1076–85.
9. Taylor S, Paluszek MM, Rachor GS, et al. Substance use and abuse, COVID-19-related distress, and disregard for social distancing: A network analysis. Addict Behav 2021;114. https://doi.org/10.1016/j.addbeh.2020.106754.
10. Lundahl LH, Cannoy C. COVID-19 and Substance Use in Adolescents. Pediatr Clin North Am 2021;68(5):977–90.
11. Roberts A, Rogers J, Mason R, et al. Alcohol and other substance use during the COVID-19 pandemic: A systematic review. Drug Alcohol Depend 2021;229:109150.
12. Pelham WE, Tapert SF, Gonzalez MR, et al. Early Adolescent Substance Use Before and During the COVID-19 Pandemic: A Longitudinal Survey in the ABCD Study Cohort. J Adolesc Health 2021;69(3):390–7.

13. Sarvey D, Welsh JW. Adolescent substance use: Challenges and opportunities related to COVID-19. J Subst Abuse Treat 2021;122.

14. Meherali S, Punjani N, Louie-Poon S, et al. Mental Health of Children and Adolescents Amidst COVID-19 and Past Pandemics: A Rapid Systematic Review. Int J Environ Res Public Health 2021;18(7). https://doi.org/10.3390/IJERPH18073432.

15. Guessoum SB, Lachal J, Radjack R, et al. Adolescent psychiatric disorders during the COVID-19 pandemic and lockdown. Psychiatry Res 2020;291.

16. Jones EAK, Mitra AK, Bhuiyan AR. Impact of COVID-19 on Mental Health in Adolescents: A Systematic Review. Int J Environ Res Public Health 2021;18(5):1–9.

17. Hawk K, D'Onofrio G. Emergency department screening and interventions for substance use disorders. Addiction Sci Clin Pract 2018;13(1):18.

18. Tuli R, Romero SA, Figueroa C, et al. Investigating a Substance Abuse Screening in a Trauma Setting. Am Surg 2021;87(10):1606–11.

19. Alcohol screening in the emergency department. Ann Emerg Med 2005;46(2):214–5.

20. SAUNDERS JB, AASLAND OG, BABOR TF, et al. Development of the Alcohol Use Disorders Identification Test (AUDIT): WHO Collaborative Project on Early Detection of Persons with Harmful Alcohol Consumption–II. Addiction 1993;88(6):791–804.

21. Bush K, Kivlahan DR, McDonell MB, et al. The AUDIT alcohol consumption questions (AUDIT-C): an effective brief screening test for problem drinking. Ambulatory Care Quality Improvement Project (ACQUIP). Alcohol Use Disorders Identification Test. Arch Intern Med 1998;158(16):1789–95.

22. Ewing JA. Detecting alcoholism. The CAGE questionnaire. JAMA 1984;252(14):1905–7.

23. O'Brien CP. The CAGE questionnaire for detection of alcoholism: a remarkably useful but simple tool. JAMA 2008;300(17):2054–6.

24. Institute on Alcohol Abuse N. Helping Patients Who Drink Too Much: A CLINICIAN'S GUIDE.

25. Smith PC, Schmidt SM, Allensworth-Davies D, et al. A single-question screening test for drug use in primary care. Arch Intern Med 2010;170(13):1155–60.

26. Morley KI, Ferris JA, Winstock AR, et al. Polysubstance use and misuse or abuse of prescription opioid analgesics: A multi-level analysis of international data. Pain 2017;158(6):1138–44.

27. El-Guebaly N. Alcohol and polysubstance abuse among women. Can J Psychiatr 1995;40(2):73–9.

28. Ogbu UC, Lotfipour S, Chakravarthy B. Polysubstance abuse: Alcohol, opioids and benzodiazepines require coordinated engagement by society, patients, and physicians. West J Emerg Med 2015;16(1):76–9.

29. GOSSOP M, GRIFFITHS P, POWIS B, et al. Severity of dependence and route of administration of heroin, cocaine and amphetamines. Br J Addict 1992;87(11):1527–36.

30. O'Donnell J, Gladden RM, Mattson CL, et al. Vital Signs: Characteristics of Drug Overdose Deaths Involving Opioids and Stimulants — 24 States and the District of Columbia, January–June 2019. MMWR Morb Mortal Wkly Rep 2020;69(35):1189–97.

31. Newcomb ME, Hill R, Buehler K, et al. High Burden of Mental Health Problems, Substance Use, Violence, and Related Psychosocial Factors in Transgender, Non-Binary, and Gender Diverse Youth and Young Adults. Arch Sex Behav 2020;49(2):645–59.

32. Turner WC, Muck RD, Muck RJ, et al. Co-occurring disorders in the adolescent mental health and substance abuse treatment systems. J Psychoactive Drugs 2004;36(4):455–62.

33. Kessler RC, Wai TC, Demler O, et al. Prevalence, severity, and comorbidity of 12-month DSM-IV disorders in the National Comorbidity Survey Replication. Arch Gen Psychiatry 2005;62(6):617–27.

34. Moeller KE, Kissack JC, Atayee RS, et al. Clinical Interpretation of Urine Drug Tests: What Clinicians Need to Know About Urine Drug Screens. Mayo Clin Proc 2017;92(5):774–96.

35. Rouse BA. Epidemiology of illicit and abused drugs in the general population, emergency department drug-related episodes, and arrestees. Clin Chem 1996; 42:1330–6.

36. Hser YI, Maglione M, Boyle K. Validity of self-report of drug use among STD patients, ER patients, and arrestees. Am J Drug Alcohol Abuse 1999;25(1):81–91.

37. Rockett IRH, Putnam SL, Jia H, et al. Declared and undeclared substance use among emergency department patients: A population-based study. Addiction 2006;101(5):706–12.

38. Chen WJ, Fang CC, Shyu RS, et al. Underreporting of illicit drug use by patients at emergency departments as revealed by two-tiered urinalysis. Addict Behav 2006;31(12):2304–8.

39. Perrone J, de Roos F, Jayaraman S, et al. Drug screening versus history in detection of substance use in ED psychiatric patients. AJEM (Am J Emerg Med) 2001; 19(1):49–51.

40. Drug Screening in the ED: Medical Legal Concerns and Applicability. ED Legal Letter. Published online 2008. Available at: https://www.reliasmedia.com/articles/14447-drug-screening-in-the-ed-medical-legal-concerns-and-applicability. Accessed November 29, 2022.

41. Stellpflug SJ, Cole JB, Greller HA. Urine Drug Screens in the Emergency Department: The Best Test May Be No Test at All. J Emerg Nurs 2020;46(6):923–31.

42. Nelson ZJ, Stellpflug SJ, Engebretsen KM. What Can a Urine Drug Screening Immunoassay Really Tell Us? J Pharm Pract 2016;29(5):516–26.

43. Saitman A, Park HD, Fitzgerald RL. False-positive interferences of common urine drug screen immunoassays: A review. J Anal Toxicol 2014;38(7):387–96.

44. Brahm NC, Yeager LL, Fox MD, et al. Commonly prescribed medications and potential false-positive urine drug screens. Am J Health Syst Pharm 2010;67(16): 1344–50.

45. Atasoy A, Daglioglu N, Gören İE, et al. Determination of synthetic cannabinoids in randomly urine samples collected from probationers in Turkey. Forensic Sci Int 2021;322. https://doi.org/10.1016/j.forsciint.2021.110752.

46. Verstraete AG. Detection Times of Drugs of Abuse in Blood, Urine, and Oral Fluid. Ther Drug Monit 2004;26:200–5.

47. Akosile W, McDermott BM. Use of the urine drug screen in psychiatry emergency service. Australas Psychiatr 2015;23(2):128–31.

48. Tenenbein M. Do you really need that emergency drug screen? Clin Toxicol 2009; 47(4):286–91.

49. N.D., no. 2006 ND 127 6/5/06. Ballensky v. Flattum-Riemers. Published online 2006.

50. Prom-Wormley EC, Ebejer J, Dick DM, et al. The genetic epidemiology of substance use disorder: A review. Drug Alcohol Depend 2017;180:241–59.

51. Tsuang MT, Bar JL, Harley RM, et al. The Harvard Twin Study of Substance Abuse: What we have learned. Harv Rev Psychiatry 2001;9(6):267–79.

52. Kendler KS, Karkowski LM, Neale MC, et al. Illicit psychoactive substance use, heavy use, abuse, and dependence in a US population-based sample of male twins. Arch Gen Psychiatry 2000;57(3):261–9.

53. Agrawal A, Lynskey MT. The genetic epidemiology of cannabis use, abuse and dependence. Addiction 2006;101:801–12.

54. Dube SR, Felitti VJ, Dong M, et al. Childhood abuse, neglect, and household dysfunction and the risk of illicit drug use: The adverse childhood experiences study. Pediatrics 2003;111(3):564–72.

55. Leza L, Siria S, López-Goñi JJ, et al. Adverse childhood experiences (ACEs) and substance use disorder (SUD): A scoping review. Drug Alcohol Depend 2021; 221:108563.

56. Felitti VJ, Anda RF, Nordenberg D, et al. Relationship of childhood abuse and household dysfunction to many of the leading causes of death in adults. The Adverse Childhood Experiences (ACE) Study. Am J Prev Med 1998;14(4): 245–58. S0749379798000178 [pii].

57. Petruccelli K, Davis J, Berman T. Adverse childhood experiences and associated health outcomes: A systematic review and meta-analysis. Child Abuse Negl 2019;97. https://doi.org/10.1016/j.chiabu.2019.104127.

58. Saunders JB. Substance use and addictive disorders in DSM-5 and ICD 10 and the draft ICD 11. Curr Opin Psychiatry 2017;30(4):227–37.

59. del Barrio V. Diagnostic and statistical manual of mental disorders. In: The curated reference collection in neuroscience and biobehavioral psychology. 5th edition; 2016. https://doi.org/10.1016/B978-0-12-809324-5.05530-9.

60. Degenhardt L, Charlson F, Ferrari A, et al. The global burden of disease attributable to alcohol and drug use in 195 countries and territories, 1990–2016: a systematic analysis for the Global Burden of Disease Study 2016. Lancet Psychiatr 2018;5(12):987–1012.

61. Hasin DS, Stinson FS, Ogburn E, et al. Prevalence, correlates, disability, and co-morbidity of DSM-IV alcohol abuse and dependence in the United States: Results from the national epidemiologic survey on alcohol and related conditions. Arch Gen Psychiatry 2007;64(7):830–42.

62. Nestler EJ. Is there a common molecular pathway for addiction? Nat Neurosci 2005;8(11):1445–9.

63. Mitchell JM, O'Neil JP, Janabi M, et al. Alcohol consumption induces endogenous opioid release in the human orbitofrontal cortex and nucleus accumbens. Sci Transl Med 2012;4(116). https://doi.org/10.1126/scitranslmed.3002902.

64. Morris PLP, Hopwood M, Whelan G, et al. Naltrexone for alcohol dependence: A randomized controlled trial. Addiction 2001;96(11):1565–73.

65. O'Malley SS, Corbin WR, Leeman RF, et al. Reduction of alcohol drinking in young adults by naltrexone: A double-blind, placebo-controlled, randomized clinical trial of efficacy and safety. J Clin Psychiatry 2015;76:e207–13.

66. O'Malley SS, Krishnan-Sarin S, Farren C, et al. Naltrexone decreases craving and alcohol self-administration in alcohol-dependent subjects and activates the hypothalamo-pituitary-adrenocortical axis. Psychopharmacology (Berl) 2002; 160(1):19–29.

67. Ray LA, Hutchison KE. Effects of naltrexone on alcohol sensitivity and genetic moderators of medication response: a double-blind placebo-controlled study. Arch Gen Psychiatry 2007;64(9):1069–77.

68. Drobes DJ, Anton RF, Thomas SE, et al. Effects of naltrexone and nalmefene on subjective response to alcohol among non-treatment-seeking alcoholics and social drinkers. Alcohol Clin Exp Res 2004;28(9):1362–70.

69. Volpicelli JR, Alterman AI, Hayashida M, et al. Naltrexone in the Treatment of Alcohol Dependence. Arch Gen Psychiatry 1992;49(11):876–80.

70. O'malley SS, Jaffe AJ, Chang G, et al. Naltrexone and Coping Skills Therapy for Alcohol Dependence: A Controlled Study. Arch Gen Psychiatry 1992;49(11): 881–7.

71. Anton RF, O'Malley SS, Ciraulo DA, et al. Combined Pharmacotherapies and Behavioral Interventions for Alcohol Dependence: The COMBINE Study: A Randomized Controlled Trial. JAMA 2006;295(17):2003–17.

72. Garbutt JC, Kranzler HR, O'Malley SS, et al. Efficacy and tolerability of long-acting injectable naltrexone for alcohol dependence: A randomized controlled trial. JAMA 2005;293(13):1617–25.

73. Johnson BA. Naltrexone long-acting formulation in the treatment of alcohol dependence. Ther Clin Risk Manag 2007;3(5):741–9. Available at: https://pubmed-ncbi-nlm-nih-gov.ezaccess.libraries.psu.edu/18472999/. Accessed November 29, 2022.

74. Olive M. Editorial [Hot topic: Pharmacotherapies for Alcoholism: The Old and the New (Guest Editor: M. Foster Olive)]. CNS Neurol Disord: Drug Targets 2012; 9(1):2–4.

75. Mason BJ, Heyser CJ. The neurobiology, clinical efficacy and safety of acamprosate in the treatment of alcohol dependence. Expert Opin Drug Saf 2010;9(1): 177–88.

76. Mason B, Heyser C. Acamprosate: A Prototypic Neuromodulator in the Treatment of Alcohol Dependence. CNS Neurol Disord: Drug Targets 2012;9(1):23–32.

77. Kampman KM, Pettinati HM, Lynch KG, et al. Initiating acamprosate within-detoxification versus post-detoxification in the treatment of alcohol dependence. Addict Behav 2009;34(6–7):581–6.

78. Paille FM, Guelfi JD, Perkins AC, et al. Double-blind randomized multicentre trial of acamprosate in maintaining abstinence from alcohol. Alcohol Alcohol 1995; 30(2):239–47.

79. Jonas DE, Amick HR, Feltner C, et al. Pharmacotherapy for Adults With Alcohol Use Disorders in Outpatient Settings: A Systematic Review and Meta-analysis. JAMA 2014;311(18):1889–900.

80. Garbutt JC, West SL, Carey TS, et al. Pharmacological treatment: Of alcohol dependence - A review of the evidence. JAMA 1999;281(14):1318–25.

81. Fuller RK, Branchey L, Brightwell DR, et al. Disulfiram Treatment of Alcoholism: A Veterans Administration Cooperative Study. JAMA, J Am Med Assoc 1986; 256(11):1449–55.

82. Perry EC. Inpatient management of acute alcohol withdrawal syndrome. CNS Drugs 2014;28(5):401–10.

83. Lindsay DL, Freedman K, Jarvis M, et al. Executive Summary of the American Society of Addiction Medicine (ASAM) Clinical Practice Guideline on Alcohol Withdrawal Management. J Addict Med 2020;14(5):376–92.

84. Wallace MS, Papp A. Opioid withdrawal. In: Anitescu M, Benzon HT, Wallace MS, editors. Challenging cases and complication management in pain medicine. Cham: Springer; 2017. p. 15–20.

85. Shah M, Huecker M. Opioid Withdrawal. StatPearls. Published 2022. Available at: https://www.ncbi.nlm.nih.gov/books/NBK526012/:Accessed November 29, 2022.

86. D'Onofrio G, Chawarski MC, O'Connor PG, et al. Emergency Department-Initiated Buprenorphine for Opioid Dependence with Continuation in Primary Care: Outcomes During and After Intervention. J Gen Intern Med 2017;32(6): 660–6.

87. Klein JW. Pharmacotherapy for Substance Use Disorders. Med Clin 2016;100(4): 891–910.
88. National Survey on Drug Use and Health. Available at: https://www.samhsa.gov/data/data-we-collect/nsduh-national-survey-drug-use-and-health.   Accessed December 1, 2022.
89. Deas D, May K, Randall C, et al. Naltrexone treatment of adolescent alcoholics: an open-label pilot study. J Child Adolesc Psychopharmacol 2005;15(5):723–8.
90. Woody GE, Poole SA, Subramaniam G, et al. Extended vs short-term buprenorphine-naloxone for treatment of opioid-addicted youth: a randomized trial. JAMA 2008;300(17):2003–11.
91. Fishman MJ, Winstanley EL, Curran E, et al. Treatment of opioid dependence in adolescents and young adults with extended release naltrexone: preliminary case-series and feasibility. Addiction 2010;105(9):1669–76.

Physiologic Effects of Substance Use

Brian Patrick Murray, DO[a],*, Emily Anne Kiernan, DO[b,c]

KEYWORDS

- Substance use • Physiologic effects of substances • Toxicity • Mechanism of action
- Substance induced psychosis

KEY POINTS

- A careful history and physical examination can help identify specific toxidromes.
- Laboratory studies rarely can help identify the substance of concern in a clinically relevant time frame but may help identify underlying end-organ effects from substance use.
- Benzodiazepines are always beneficial in agitation from substance use but may require high doses.
- For any clinical concerns, a local poison center is always available for consultation at 1-800-222-1222.

INTRODUCTION

Complications from substance use have increased year after year, with an estimated 107,622 deaths from overdose in 2021, an increase of 15% from 93,655 in 2022.[1] In 2017, US Emergency Department and inpatient costs related to substance use disorder exceeded $13 billion dollars.[2] While mu-receptor agonists, in particular fentanyl, amphetamines, and cocaine make up most of the deaths and discussion about substance use,[1] there is a large number of drug classes that are abused, ranging from readily available household substances to legally available drugs. Each drug carries its own risk of addiction, withdrawal, and physiologic effects. Even among each individual drug, the effects can vary dramatically depending on the formulation and route of administration.

Reasons for substance use are as varied as the substances used. Drugs can provide an escape from reality, euphoric experience, altered the perception of reality, or a different understanding of the world. Differences are based on the site of action or the direct or indirect receptor interactions with each drug. People frequently initiate

[a] Department of Emergency Medicine, Wright State Boonshoft School of Medicine, 2555 University Boulevard, Suite 110, Dayton, OH 45324, USA; [b] Department of Emergency Medicine, Emory University School of Medicine, 50 Hurtz Plaza Southeast, Suite 600, Atlanta, GA, USA; [c] Georgia Poison Center, 50 Hurtz Plaza Southeast, Suite 600, Atlanta, GA, USA
* Corresponding author.
E-mail address: brian.murray@wright.edu

Emerg Med Clin N Am 42 (2024) 69–91
https://doi.org/10.1016/j.emc.2023.06.022
0733-8627/24/Published by Elsevier Inc.

emed.theclinics.com

substance use for a euphoric experience, which is tied to increased dopamine activity in the mesolimbic system. Dopamine highjacks the reward system of the brain, leading to addiction and drug seeking behavior. While substance use may begin for a pleasurable experience, eventually one's neurocircuitry can be reorganized through tolerance and neuroadaptation and eventually use becomes more about preventing withdrawal than obtaining a pleasurable experience.

Not all drugs have the same addictive potential. Drugs that have an increased or oversized effect on dopamine in the limbic system, drugs that are rapidly absorbed into the blood and into the brain, and drugs with a short duration of action all increase the likelihood of chemical addiction. While conversely, drugs with a slower absorption, less rapid brain penetration, and longer metabolism or elimination half-life are protective against addiction. Additionally, drugs that have little effect on the dopaminergic reward system are also less likely to result in chemical addiction. Although psychological addiction is still possible.

The association between substance use disorder and psychiatric illness is complex. Among patients with opioid use disorder, approximately 65% have a co-occurring mental illness, and 27% have a serious mental illness.[3] There is also a strong connection between major depressive episodes and illicit drug use in general as well as with marijuana, binge alcohol, and cigarette use.[4] There is a significant overlap between patients with psychiatric illness and substance use disorder, but whether one influences the other, or whether there is an unconscious attempt at self-treatment is not well understood.

In this article we will explore the physiologic effects of common drugs of abuse. In each section, we will review the mechanism of action of each drug or drug class, the intoxicated state, potential withdrawal state, and long-term medical and psychiatric consequences associated with use.

Ethanol

Ethanol is one of the oldest mind-altering substances used by humans. Residue found on 9000-year-old pottery provides evidence that ethanol was consumed as far back as the neolithic age.[5] It has a dose-dependent action, initially decreasing inhibition and enhancing sociability, but at higher doses producing ataxia, central nervous system (CNS) depression, and respiratory depression.

Ethanol primarily works through agonism of the γ-aminobutyric acid-A receptor (GABA-Ar) in the CNS. This receptor functions as a chloride ion (Cl^-) channel, allowing for inward flow of Cl^- in the postsynaptic neuron, causing the hyperpolarization and inhibition of post-synaptic action potentials. Therefore, ethanol increases postsynaptic inhibition which is the cause of the CNS and respiratory depression in ethanol intoxication. Ethanol also interacts with the N-methyl-D-aspartate (NMDA) receptor, a glutamate reception which allows voltage controlled inward flow of calcium (Ca^{2+}), potassium (K^+), and sodium (Na^+) ions, leading to the activation of intracellular signaling pathways and hypopolarization, increasing the likelihood of further depolarization. Glutamate receptors are the major excitatory receptor in the CNS. Ethanol inhibits the NMDA receptor decreasing excitation as well as negatively modulating the control of synaptic plasticity as well as learning and memory.[6] Additionally, through NMDA inhibition, ethanol increases dopamine release in the nucleus accumbens and ventral tegmental areas, contributing to its addictive potential.

The effects of intoxication begin with a blood alcohol concentration (BAC, expressed as mg of ethanol in 100 mL) as low as 0.08%. At this concentration one would have a change in personality, increased sociability, and impairment in judgment. At levels of 0.1% to 0.3% slurred speech and ataxia become more prevalent.

At levels greater than 0.4% stupor and coma may occur. Of course, a person's tolerance will play into the exact effect at each concentration, with chronic heavy ethanol users tolerating higher concentrations. Additionally, the effect felt by alcohol is different depending on if the blood concentration is increasing or decreasing. This is called the Mallanby effect, and patients will feel more intoxicated at the same concentration if their BAC is increasing, than if it is decreasing. However, while the the perception of intoxication is decreased, judgment and motor skills are still impaired.[7]

Complications of ethanol use include hypoglycemia (particularly in pediatric patients and malnourished patients), increased sleep initiation but decreased sleep persistence, and Wernicke-Karsakoff syndrome with chronic use. Hypoglycemia results from the buildup of NADH, a byproduct of metabolism by alcohol dehydrogenase and aldehyde dehydrogenase, both of which utilize NAD^+ as a catalyst in alcohol metabolism. This imbalance of NAD^+ and NADH leads to impaired gluconeogenesis, and the conversion of pyruvate to lactic acid, as a means of regenerating NAD^+.[8] Sleep disturbances result from the agonism of GABA-A and antagonism of NMDA receptors, which as the alcohol is metabolized reverses this sedation and limits deep and restful sleep. This sleep disturbance may take several months to return to normal in chronic heavy drinkers but is short-lived in occasional drinkers.[9]

Wernicke Encephalopathy is identified as a triad of ophthalmoplegia, ataxia, and confusion. Additionally, it is typically also associated with a loss of appetite, tachycardia, and urinary retention (from anticholinergic autonomic dysfunction), and may be confused with acute withdrawal symptoms, but will persist after withdrawal as resolved. It is caused by a thiamine deficiency, typically from poor nutrition in chronic alcohol users. While Karsakoff syndrome, also from thiamine deficiency, results in confabulation due to severe anterograde, and to a lesser extent retrograde, amnesia. Treatment is with high dose thiamine replacement, and recovery may take many months. Patients may not recover fully, and some degree of ataxia and dementia may be permanent.[10]

Heavy alcohol use is also associated with an increased risk of hemorrhagic strokes, Marchiafava-Binami disease (a demyelinating and necrotic disease of the CNS),[11] alcohol cardiomyopathy, and arrhythmias, particularly atrial fibrillation (holiday heart).[12,13] Electrolyte disturbances, particularly hyponatremia, arise from poor nutrition as well as increased free water intake from excessive alcohol ingestion (Beer Potomania).[14,15]

Moderate drinking is defined as equal to or less than 2 drinks daily for men and one drink daily for women. Heavy, at-risk, drinking is defined by the National Institute on Alcohol Abuse and Alcoholism (NIAAA) as consuming 4 or more drinks on any 1 day and more than 14 drinks in a week for men and consuming 3 or more drinks on any 1 day or more than 7 drinks per week for women. The Substance Abuse and Mental Health Services Administration (SAMHSA) defines heavy drinking as binge drinking on 5 or more days in the past month. Binge drinking is defined as a pattern of drinking that brings the BAC to greater than 0.08%, which is approximately 5 or more drinks for men, and 4 or more drinks for women in a 2-hour period.[16] A drink is defined as 15 gm, or 0.6 oz, of pure ethanol. This is typically found in a 12 oz beer or cooler (5% ethanol v/v), 5 oz wine (12% ethanol v/v), or 1.5 oz spirits (40% ethanol v/v).

While heavy drinking and at-risk drinking are risk factors for developing alcohol use disorder (AUD), not everyone who exhibits at risk drinking behavior will develop AUD (**Box 1**).[17,18] However, even without a formal diagnosis of AUD, patients may exhibit withdrawal symptoms when they stop drinking. There are distinct alcohol withdrawal syndromes and the symptoms do not have to occur in a stepwise fashion and may happen in any order.

Box 1
DSM-V alcohol user disorder criteria[66]

Had times when you ended up drinking more, or longer, than you intended?

More than once wanted to cut down or stop drinking, or tried to, but couldn't?

Spent a lot of time drinking? Or being sick or getting over other aftereffects?

Wanted a drink so badly you couldn't think of anything else?

Found that drinking—or being sick from drinking—often interfered with taking care of your home or family? Or caused job troubles? Or school problems?

Continued to drink even though it was causing trouble with your family or friends?

Given up or cut back on activities that were important or interesting to you, or gave you pleasure, in order to drink?

More than once gotten into situations while or after drinking that increased your chances of getting hurt (such as driving, swimming, using machinery, walking in a dangerous area, or having unsafe sex)?

Continued to drink even though it was making you feel depressed or anxious or adding to another health problem? Or after having had a memory blackout?

Had to drink much more than you once did to get the effect you want? Or found that your usual number of drinks had much less effect than before?

Found that when the effects of alcohol were wearing off, you had withdrawal symptoms, such as trouble sleeping, shakiness, restlessness, nausea, sweating, a racing heart, or a seizure? Or sensed things that were not there?

The presence of at least 2 of these symptoms indicatesAlcohol Use Disorder (AUD).The severity of the AUD is defined as: Mild: The presence of 2 to 3 symptoms; Moderate: The presence of 4 to 5 symptoms; Severe: The presence of 6 or more symptoms.

Autonomic hyperactivity is characterized by tremors, anxiety, diaphoresis, insomnia, and nausea and vomiting, but with a clear sensorium. Onset is typically within 6 hours after the last drink, and peaks at 24 to 48 hours. Hallucinations, which are typically visual, but may also be auditory and tactile, can last up to 6 days after the last drink. Seizures may also occur in up to 10% of individuals and most commonly will occur 12 to 48 hours after the last drink, but in some individuals, they can occur earlier, and in severe chronic alcohol use, may even occur before the alcohol fully clears. About 50% of patients who develop alcohol withdrawal seizures will have more than one seizure and 5% will develop status epilepticus. Seizures independently increase the risk of death by approximately 4-fold independent of the risks from the seizure itself but are a surrogate for the severity of the withdrawal. Delirium tremens (DT) occurs 48 to 72 hours after the last drink and is characterized by acute delirium, most commonly hyperactive but it may also be hypoactive. DTs can last up to 14 days postingestion and is also a marker of severe withdrawal and is associated with a worse prognosis.[19]

AUD has a complex relationship with multiple psychiatric illnesses and patients with AUD have a higher prevalence of mood, anxiety, thought, and other substance use disorders. There is approximately a 3.5 to 4 hazard ratio for having a cooccurring substance use disorder. Major depressive disorder has an odds ratio of about 2-3x for to co-occur with AUD, and anxiety disorders have an odds ratio of about 1.5 to 1.6x co-occurrence with AUD.[20] While many of these individuals may have an underlying depression or anxiety disorder that they are attempting to self-treat with alcohol,

alcohol itself has the ability to cause depression with up to about 25% of patients with any substance induced depression experiencing a substance induced depressive episode.[21] The mechanism underlying this induced depression is not understood. This is an important concept to understand as it has implications for the most appropriate treatment modalities. Patients with underlying depression, or any psychiatric disorder, will benefit from psychiatric treatment in conjunction with treatment for their substance use, while patients with substance induced depression will improve with abstinence and may not require further medical management of the co-occurring psychiatric condition. Although, there is thought that while the immediate depression resolves with the cessation of use, these patients may be at risk of developing major depressive disorder later in life.[22]

Additionally, alcohol use and AUD both influence the rate of suicide. In a meta-analysis of 30 articles, there was a significant association between the use of alcohol and attempted and completed suicide, with a relative ratio of 1.65.[23] In a Swedish study, AUD was associated with a lifetime risk of suicide of 3.54% for women and 3.95% for men, with a baseline population rate of suicide of 0.29% and 0.76% for women and men respectively.[24]

There are nearly 14.5 million adults, aged 12 and older, who were diagnosed with AUD in 2019.[25] The annual mortality, from 2011 to 2015, was 95,158 people from alcohol-related causes in the US.[26] Unfortunately, a minute fraction of people with AUD receive treatment. Of those that do, most will have at least some recurrence of drinking within a 5 to 10-year time frame. For patients that develop secondary and tertiary complications, many will have long-term disability, some severe with permanent disability. An understanding of the pathophysiology and complications of alcohol use is important to counsel patients and initiate treatment when indicated.

Sedative Hypnotics (Barbiturates, Benzodiazepines, Z-drugs)

Sedative hypnotics make up a class of drugs whose main effect is agonism of the γ-aminobutyric acid-A receptor (GABA-Ar). The end effect is psycholepsis, anxiolysis, sedation, sleep initiation, muscle relaxation, cessation of seizurogenic activity, and amnesia. The GABA-Ar is an ionotropic receptor and ligand-gated ion channel. The endogenous ligand is γ-aminobutyric acid (GABA), the primary inhibitory neurotransmitter of the central nervous system (CNS). The 3 types of drugs that make up the sedative hypnotic drug class are barbiturates, benzodiazepines, and the newer "Z-drugs" which are non-benzodiazepines that have activity at the same site on the GABA-Ar as benzodiazepines.

The GABA-Ar protein consists of 5 subunits arranged around a central pore. While all receptors must possess an α and β subunit, most commonly the configuration contains 2 α and 2 β subunits, frequently associated with a γ subunit. The primary ion that passes through the channel, when activated, is a chloride (Cl^-) ion, which flows into the cell hyperpolarizing the membrane potential. Although the direction of the ion flow is dependent on the chemical gradient and in some instances can be reversed.

The benzodiazepine (as well as z-drug and flumazenil) binding site is between the α and γ subunits, while the GABA allosteric site is between the α and β subunits. The barbiturate binding site is a distinct site from the benzodiazepine site. There are numerous configurations possible, and the receptors with α1-, α2-, α3-, or α5-are all benzodiazepine sensitive. While receptors with α4-, or α6-subunits may be resistant to some benzodiazepines.[27] This can become problematic in severe chronic ethanol and benzodiazepine use as there may be a subunit type change in response to chronic use and tolerance.[28]

Barbiturates were the first subclass discovered in 1864 with the discover of barbituric acid, the basic core structure of all barbiturates, which doesn't have any activity at the GABA-A receptor. However, barbiturates weren't recognized as a useful pharmaceutical drug until 1903 when barbital, the first true barbiturate, was noted to put dogs to sleep. It was used for nearly 50 years until its dependence potential was noted until 1950.

Barbiturates work by modulating the activity of the GABAr. At low doses, they allow the receptor to stay open for a longer time period when the channel is activated by the GABA, but do not themselves open the chloride channel. However, at high doses, barbiturates can open the ion channel independent of GABA. This allows for severe toxicity in overdose, producing profound CNS and respiratory depression.

In addition to their activity at the GABA-Ar, barbiturates also inhibit the AMPA receptor, a glutamate reception which allows voltage controlled inward flow of calcium (Ca^{2+}), potassium (K^+), and sodium (Na^+) ions. Additionally, at high concentrations, barbiturates can inhibit Ca^{2+}-dependent release of glutamate. In addition to the lack of a ceiling effect, the antagonism of AMPA and inhibition of glutamate release contribute to the profound CNS depression experienced with barbiturates. There is no reversal agent for barbiturate overdose.

Benzodiazepines were first discovered in 1955, with the accidental synthesis of chlordiazepoxide, followed closely by diazepam in 1963. Benzodiazepines are based on the fusion of a benzene right to a diazepine ring. Owing to their "clean" mechanism of action, in that they are specific for the GABA-Ar, and their safer profile in overdose, they quickly became one of the most prescribed medications globally, replacing the more dangerous barbiturates.

Unlike barbiturates, which increase the duration the GABA-Ar ion channel is open, benzodiazepines increase the frequency of ion channel opening in the presence of GABA and are unable to open the ion channel independent of GABA, regardless of concentration. This modulation is due to positive allosteric modulation, their binding to the GABA-Ar changes the receptor conformation such that there is an increased capacity to bind GABA[28] and creates a strong ceiling effect where, in overdose, once all the GABA-Ar are bound to benzodiazepines, no further sedation is possible. Additionally, even after large overdoses, single agent ingestions of benzodiazepines are not associated with respiratory depression. This does not hold true if the is co-ingestion of another CNS or respiratory depressant such as alcohol or a mu-opioid receptor agonist.

All benzodiazepines have comparable pharmacodynamic activity, but primarily differ in their pharmacokinetic activity. The mode of administration, rate of absorption, time to peak effect, duration of action, and elimination half-life vary from drug to drug, and this is the primary consideration when deciding on which medication to prescribe.

The "Z-drugs" are newer non-benzodiazepine medications that bind to the same allosteric site on the GABA-Ar. They are termed Z-drugs because the names of the first drugs in this class start with the letter "Z" (eg, zolpidem, zaleplon, zopiclone). As they bind to the same allosteric site as benzodiazepines, they have all the same effects as benzodiazepines. They were thought to have a decreased risk of dependence when compared to benzodiazepines.[29] However, the risk may be higher than initially anticipated,[30] and they may have a higher adverse effect profile.[31] There is cross-tolerance with benzodiazepines.

Unfortunately, benzodiazepines do have abuse potential. Part of this comes from rapid tolerance to the psycholepsis, requiring escalating doses and physical dependence.[32] They also influence the dopamine in the mesolimbic pathway, just as all addictive drugs do.[33] However, unlike most other drugs, except other GABA receptor modulators, withdrawal can be dangerous, and even life threatening. Due to an insufficient amount of GABA inhibition from down-regulation of receptors, and subunit compositional changes, affected individuals may undergo seizure activity that may be difficult to control.[32]

Single-time dosing of benzodiazepines in the Emergency Department for agitated individuals will not increase the risk of dependence or sedative hypnotic use disorder. Starting a prescription from the ED for more than several doses, such as a short course of diazepam for muscle relaxation, can be a concern in some individuals who have a predisposition to developing a use disorder. However, individuals who are chronically on benzodiazepines who require a refill are more complicated. The physician will need to balance the risk of continued use and feeding into a system where the patient feels it appropriate to come to the Emergency Department for refills of controlled substances against a potentially life-threatening withdrawal, possibly causing the patient to look to street drugs which may be laced with other non-benzodiazepine sedatives, including fentanyl, to prevent withdrawal. The best course of action is to have a frank conversation about the concerns over long-term use, dependence, and the lack of benefit long-term from these agents, and help connect them to resources that can help taper them down. Unfortunately, it can take months of taper benzodiazepines to safely stop using them, a time frame not available in an Emergency Department setting.

Flumazenil is a GABA-Ar antagonist that blocks the action of both benzodiazepines and Z-drugs. While flumazenil can reverse the CNS depression caused by benzodiazepines, in patients who chronically take a benzodiazepine and have tolerance, antagonist can induce severe withdrawal and seizures.[34] This risk is increased if the patient is on another seizure threshold-lowering medication.[35] However, despite the very real concerns over sedative hypnotic reversal leading to severe withdrawal symptoms, its use may not be as dangerous as initially thought,[36] particularly when used to reverse overaggressive procedural sedation in a benzodiazepine-naïve individual.[37] Despite this, CNS depression is not synonymous with respiratory depression, and the concern over flumazenil-precipitated withdrawal is real. Therefore great care must be taken prior to using flumazenil to reverse undifferentiated CNS depression. Ultimately, if needed, intubation and allowing the medication to metabolize might be the safest option. Interestingly, at low doses, flumazenil might have partial agonist properties, and may be useful in alleviating withdrawal symptoms in patients with benzodiazepine dependence.[38]

Cocaine

Cocaine was involved in nearly 1 in 5 overdose deaths in 2019, according to the Substance Abuse and Mental Health Services Administration (SAMHSA), and over 5 million Americans reported current cocaine use in 2020.[4]

A cocaine alkaloid is extracted from *Erythroxylum coca leaves,* a native shrub to Colombia, Peru, Bolivia, the West Indies, and Indonesia, to make a water-soluble white powder (cocaine hydrochloride), which can be insufflated, applied to mucous membranes, ingested, or injected (after dissolved in water). "Crack" is a free base form of cocaine produced by precipitating cocaine "rocks" that can be smoked.

Cocaine is used in clinical medicine as a local anesthetic (LA). Like other LAs, cocaine halts the initiation and propagation of nerve impulses by blocking the fast sodium ion channels, altering axonal membrane permeability, and halting further nerve conduction. The mechanism of action for recreational purposes results from the reuptake blockade of multiple neurotransmitters including, dopamine, serotonin, epinephrine, and norepinephrine. Dopamine is the key neuromodulator and is responsible for the desired effects including intense euphoria and elation. Cocaine increases synaptic dopaminergic concentrations by blocking the presynaptic dopamine transporter (DAT) which is responsible for reabsorbing synaptic dopamine back into the presynaptic neuron and prevents dopamine re-uptake.[39] Excessive synaptic dopamine can cause paranoia, hallucinations, and dysphoria. Patients may also experience choreoathetoid movements from dopamine depletion, often referred to as "crack dancing."[40] Serotonin plays a role as a dopamine modulator and partially antagonize the stimulatory effects of cocaine, but it also plays a role in cocaine addiction, reward, and potential seizure-activity. Excessive epinephrine and norepinephrine are responsible for the classic sympathomimetic toxidrome including, hypertension, and tachycardia, diaphoresis, mydriasis, and hyperthermia.[41]

The intoxication syndrome caused by cocaine is notable for its hyperadrenergic state and potent vasoconstriction. The most common severe clinical manifestations after acute cocaine intoxication are psychosis, seizure, ventricular arrhythmias, respiratory dysfunction, hypertension leading to hypotension, and fasciculations. Cocaine produces blockade of cardiac sodium and potassium channels resulting in QRS and QT interval prolongation and increases the risk of wide complex tachycardia and torsade de pointes, respectively.[42,43] "Crack lung" describes a pulmonary syndrome of fever, hypoxia, hemoptysis, progressing to acute respiratory distress syndrome (ARDS) and respiratory failure from direct lung injury after smoking crack and/or the associated impurities.[44] Additionally, pneumothorax or pneumomediastinum can be seen after intense insufflation. If cocaine is used with ethanol, cocaethylene, an active metabolite, is produced and can cause more euphoria, increased cardiotoxicity, and longer duration of action than cocaine intoxication alone.[45]

Cocaine withdrawal syndrome is not well defined. However, a "wash-out" syndrome occurs after acute or chronic use which correlates with a dopamine and norepinephrine depleted state. Patients may present with hypersomnolence, anergia, anhedonia, and generalized weakness with difficulty initiating and sustaining movement. However, cognitive deficits generally do not exist. Depression and anhedonia after cocaine cessation partially result from a decrease in synaptic serotonin concentrations.[46] No specific treatment exists for cocaine wash-out syndrome and supportive care should be provided.

Chronic cocaine use can lead to a variety of long-term complications and can produce end-organ toxicity in virtually every organ system secondary to vasospasm, hemorrhage, and/or enhanced coagulation.[41] Cardiovascular toxicity is the most concerning and is multifactorial[1]: exposure to high levels of catecholamines with resultant tachycardia and hypertension,[2] increased myocardial oxygen demand,[3] potent vasoconstriction with resultant coronary artery vasospasm and diminished blood flow,[4] accelerated atherogenesis, and[5] hypercoagulability, all contribute to myocardial ischemia and infarction. Cocaine-induced hyperthermia is also a life-threatening complication that can be due to the hyperadrenergic state, but also may be related to downregulated dopamine-2 receptors in the hypothalamus. Cocaine-induced hyperactive delirium with severe agitation (previously known as excited delirium), defined as hyperthermia, delirium, agitation, cardiorespiratory arrest, and sudden death, is seen in patients with acute, large exposure to cocaine.[47] Subarachnoid and intracerebral hemorrhages, berry aneurysms, cerebral infarction, and cocaine-induced seizures have all been reported in addition to cocaine-hyperactive delirium with severe agitation.[41,47] Rates of antisocial personality disorders (ASP) and mood disorders are common among people who use drugs, with ASPs typically being more common. However, in people who use cocaine, the rates of ASP and mood disorders is more equal, or with a higher rate of mood disorders. Like with ethanol, it can be very complex to tease apart how much of the mood disorder is a preexisting condition versus drug induced mood disorder. As cocaine is a serotonin reuptake inhibitor, it is wholly possibly that patients use cocaine to self-treat depression. But in doing so, they create a scenario where they further perpetuate this depression and make it worse since cocaine use can trigger or exacerbate psychological, behavioral, and mental health disorders, particularly with chronic, long-term use.[48,49]

People who receive cocaine from an unknown source must be cautious as it may be mixed with stimulant drugs (eg, amphetamines), adulterants (eg, cornstarch, talc powder, caffeine), or other illicit drugs (eg, heroin, fentanyl).[50]

Currently, the Food & Drug Administration does not have an approved medication for the treatment of cocaine use disorder, despite decades of clinical trials. However, contingency management and cognitive behavioral therapy may be used to treat patients with CUD.[51]

Amphetamines

The structure of amphetamines is a methyl homolog of the neurotransmitter phenethylamine, which regulates monoamine neurotransmission though the modulation of the trace amine-associated receptor 1 (TAAR1) and inhibiting the vesicular monoamine transporter 2 (VMAT2). The TAAR1 is an intracellular G-coupled protein that plays a critical role in the regulation dopamine, norepinephrine, dopamine, norepinephrine, and serotonin, and VMAT2 transports monoamines (dopamine, norepinephrine, serotonin, histamine) from the neuronal cytosol into a synaptic vesicle.

In 2020, 2.5 million Americans aged 12 or older reported having used methamphetamine in the past year.[4] Amphetamines are the representatives of compounds with a structural phenylethylamines backbone and are naturally found in the ephedra plant. Structurally similar drugs (eg, methamphetamine MDMA) have specific clinical effects that will not be discussed in this section. Unregulated novel synthetic cathinones have also emerged as designer drugs of abuse.

The primary mechanism of action of amphetamines involves the release of catecholamines (dopamine, norepinephrine, serotonin) from presynaptic terminals leading to a hyperadrenergic state. Amphetamines enter the neuron in a dose dependent fashion and the amount of catecholamine released is dependent on the amount of amphetamine administered.[52] The release of dopamine in the neostriatum mediates stereotypical behavior and locomotor activities, activity in neostriatum linked to glutamate release and inhibition of GABA. Serotonin release causes hallucinations, release of ADH, and regulation of fluid secretion, peristalsis, and vascular beds.[53] While the effects on dopamine and serotonin may be desired (altered perception, anorexia), it also leads to psychotic behaviors. Norepinephrine releases from the locus cerelus and leads to the desired effects of decreased fatigue and increased attentiveness, it also causes vasoconstriction and hypertension.

There are several ways in when amphetamines increase dopamine. They act, like cocaine, as a dopamine reuptake inhibitor, through competitive inhibition, of the dopamine transporter (DAT). However, instead of blocking it, they cause it to run backwards, expelling dopamine from the presynaptic cytosol into the synaptic cleft. They also act by blocking the vesicular monoamine transporter 2 (VMAT2) which transports monoamines (dopamine, norepinephrine, serotonin, histamine) from the neuronal cytosol into a synaptic vesicle. Therefore, amphetamines block dopamine reuptake, increase cytosolic dopamine by preventing sequestration in synaptic vesicles, actively move dopamine, in an unregulated fashion, from the cytosol into the synapse and have several other effects on monoamine formation and metabolism. All this means that amphetamines increase synaptic dopamine more than almost any other substance, making amphetamines incredibly addictive, and difficult to stop using.[54]

Amphetamines are rapidly absorbed by inhalation, intravenous, intramuscular, or transmucosal routes. Symptoms can last hours to days based on the dose and strength. Amphetamines are relatively lipophilic and can cross the blood brain barrier. Additionally, increased toxicity is a concern in patients with diminished CYP2D6 activity.[55]

Clinical manifestations of intoxication are associated with uncontrolled hyperadrenergic states and present with the classic sympathomimetic toxidrome of diaphoresis, mydriasis, tachypnea, tachycardia, hypertension, agitation, and tremor. Acute toxicity generally manifests with central nervous system effects (choreoathetoid movements, euphoria, headache, hyperreflexia, hyperthermia, intracerebral hemorrhage, paranoid psychosis, seizures) and cardiovascular toxicity (aortic dissection, dysrhythmias, myocardial ischemia, vasospasm).

The withdrawal syndrome of amphetamines is not well-described, but patients will develop tolerance and psychological dependence after chronic amphetamine use and may return to normal sensorium after discontinuing use. However, increased dopaminergic pathways lead to glutamate excesses in the cerebral cortex which leads to the dysregulation of glutamate in the cerebral cortex and possible psychosis.[56] Prior psychiatric studies have found that GABAergic cortical dysfunction seems to relate to schizophrenia.[57]

Patients will often experience compulsive repetitive behavior patterns during periods of use (eg, picking, bruxism, repetitive tasks). Choreoathetoid movements are caused by increased dopamine in striatal areas of the brain. Patients can also experience aortic and mitral regurgitation, cardiomyopathy, pulmonary hypertension, and vasculitis in any organ system.

Episodes of amphetamine-induced psychosis are likely to be recurrent with subsequent exposures. Amphetamine-induced psychosis is difficult to differentiate from an organic mental health illness. It is often confused for schizophrenia given the overlap with persecutory delusions, visual hallucinations, and acute psychosis. Skin picking is a common manifestation due to delusions of parasitosis. Poor oral hygiene is often seen with severe dental caries and inflamed gingiva.

Treatment consists of discontinuing the use the drug, determine the underlying cause of the patient's stimulant use, and address and treat the patient's signs and symptoms. Antipsychotics, like olanzapine and haloperidol, may be helpful resolving psychotic symptoms.[58]

While there is no specific FDA-approved treatment for amphetamine use disorder, the treatment is likely multifactorial and should include cognitive behavioral therapy or contingency management.

Marijuana

Marijuana is the common name for a mixture of dried leaves and flowers of the Cannabis sativa plant, but cannabis more broadly refers to the group of bioactive substances, or cannabinoids, from the Cannabis plant. Cannabis contains >500 different chemicals, including >109 cannabinoids; the major cannabinoids are cannabinol, cannabidiol (CBD), and tetrahydrocannabinol, with Δ9-tetrahydrocannabinol (THC) being the primary psychoactive substance. Other forms of cannabis include hashish and hashish oil (pressed resin and oil expressed from the pressed resin, respectively) which are highly concentrated products that are "dabbed" or ingested. Butane and other solvent extractions of cannabis produce highly concentrated (80%–100%) THC wax or butane hash oil (BHO). Many edible THC products are now on the market (regulated and unregulated). Unregulated synthetic cannabinoids have also emerged as designer drugs of abuse.

Humans have an endogenous cannabinoid system which plays a role in movement control, pain modulation, and memory.[59] Marijuana binds to G protein-coupled cannabinoid receptors. There are 2 main types of cannabinoid receptor: CB_1 and CB_2, distinguished largely by their anatomic distribution and mechanisms of cellular messaging. The mechanism of action for marijuana depends on the receptor stimulated. THC acts on dopaminergic projections in the brain and acts as a direct or indirect dopamine agonist in the reward circuitry in acute exposure.[60]

CB_1 and CB_2 receptors are in the CNS, with CB_1 predominating and mediate the effects of THC. CB_1 receptor are mainly located on GABA-ergic neurons in the hippocampus, amygdala, and cortex and activation can inhibit or enhance release of acetylcholine, norepinephrine, dopamine, 5-hydroxytryptamine (5-HT), γ-aminobutyric acid (GABA), and glutamate. CB_1 receptors is believed to be responsible for the clinical effects of cannabinoids, including the regulation of cognition, memory, motor activities, nociception, nausea, and vomiting.[61]

The mechanism of action and clinical effects of marijuana depends on the pharmacokinetics, route of administration, concentration of the product, frequency of use, and coexistent psychoactive drug use. Inhalation of THC-containing smoke or vaping results in a faster onset of psychoactive effects when compared to ingestion or "dabbing," which can lead to excessive ingestion of THC containing products. Additionally, marijuana is lipophilic and slowly eliminated from the body. Physiologically, marijuana increases blood flow to the cerebrum, the heart, the lungs, and the eyes. Acute intoxication with marijuana will increase heart rate and blood pressure and cause conjunctival injection. Acute toxicity can cause decreased coordination, muscle strength, and hand steadiness, lethargy, sedation, postural hypotension (due to decreased systemic vascular resistance), inability to concentrate, decreased psychomotor activity, slurred speech, and slow reaction time.

An intoxication syndrome occurs at high doses and can manifest as panic reactions, paranoia, hallucinations, illusions, thought disorganization, agitation, and transient psychosis with depersonalization and loss of insight. This can exacerbate preexisting psychiatric disease. Interestingly, formulations with a higher ratio of CBD:THC are less psychosis-associated with use.[62] Toxicity in children can be more pronounced with tachycardia or bradycardia, obtundation, apnea, cyanosis, and hypotonia.

The effects of synthetic cannabinoids have not been well described given variations in nomenclature and unregulated products.[63] As a class, they are described as more potent with increased physiologic effects versus traditional cannabis. Additionally, products may be adulterated or be sold as a "spice" blends or incense, making it difficult to understand the underlying pathophysiology and clinical effects. These agents bind more strongly to cannabinoid receptors producing an exaggerated stimulant effect, with severe aggression and psychosis reported.[64]

Multiple daily THC exposures over an extended period of time are needed to develop tolerance to the behavioral and physiologic effects of cannabis, however, it tends to be less pronounced.[59,65] Cannabis withdrawal syndrome is described as 3 of the following symptoms within 7 days of reduced cannabis use[1]: irritability, anger, or aggression[2]; nervousness or anxiety[3]; sleep disturbance[4]; appetite or weight disturbance[5]; restlessness[6]; depressed mood; and[7] somatic symptoms, such as headaches, sweating, nausea, vomiting, or abdominal pain.[66] CWS may be more common in patients with comorbid drug or tobacco use or more frequent and potent cannabis use but tends to be short-lived and less pronounced than other drug withdrawal states. The amount, frequency, and duration of marijuana use required to develop dependence are not well established and support for cannabis dependence is based on the existence of a withdrawal syndrome.[67] Another described state in patients with chronic cannabis use is amotivational syndrome with apathy, underachievement, and lack of energy.[68]

Research regarding chronic cannabis use and deficits in cognition and learning are ongoing, however, the current evidence does not strongly support these findings. However, patients with cannabis use at a younger age, use of potent cannabinoids, and those with underlying psychiatric disorders are more likely to exhibit psychotic features are cannabinoid exposure.[59] Treatment of cannabis use disorder is challenging because there are no efficacious medications available, despite marketed cannabinoid replacement therapies.

Opioids

Overdoses involving opioids killed nearly 69,000 people in the United States in 2020, and over 82% of those deaths involved synthetic opioids. Opiates (morphine, codeine) are naturally derived from opium poppy, *Papaver somniferum,* whereas opioids are semisynthetic (heroin, oxycodone) or synthetic (methadone, meperidine) and produce an opium-like effect or binds to an opioid receptor. Endogenous opioids (β—endorphin, enkephalins, and dynorphin) are distributed throughout the brain and modulate responses to painful stimuli, stressors, reward, and homeostatic adaptive functions via a nondopaminergic system of opioid reward. The ventral tegmental area, nucleus accumbens, hippocampus, and hypothalamus are responsible, in part, for reinforcing and rewarding effects of opioids. Unregulated novel synthetic opioids have also emerged as designer drugs of abuse.

The mechanism of action for opioids depends on which receptors are stimulated. There are 3 main types of opioid receptor: μ, δ, and κ, herein described as MOP, KOP, and DOP, respectively, which are all G protein-coupled receptors. The mechanism of action for opioids depends on the receptors that are stimulated. MOP is the morphine binding site. MOP1 receptors are concentrated in the brain and involved in analgesia (periaqueductal gray, nucleus raphe magnus, medial thalamus), euphoria and reward (mesolimbic system), respiratory function (medulla). MOP2 produces spinal level analgesia but can also cause respiratory depression. KOP is a dysnorphin binding site that produces spinal analgesia, miosis, diuresis, without respiratory depression or constipation. DOP is an enkephalin binding site that is important in spinal and supraspinal analgesia and cough suppression but may also modulate dopamine release and play a role in behavioral reinforcement.[69]

The desired effect of an opioid depends on the formulation and the targeted receptor. Analgesia is achieved by modulating cerebral cortical pain perception at supraspinal, spinal, and peripheral levels. Dopamine release from the mesolimbic system causes the desired euphoric effects.[70] N-methyl-D-aspartate (NMDA) receptor blockade can also enhance the analgesic effects of MOP agonists.[71]

The clinical intoxication of opioids affects multiple systems. Opioid toxidrome consists of respiratory depression, central nervous system depression, and miosis. After an overdose, patients will present with diminished ventilatory effort or apnea due to the loss of the hypercarbic stimulation to breath with resultant hypercarbia and hypoxia. Acute respiratory distress syndrome (ARDS) has been described after prolonged respiratory depression and reversal by the antidote, naloxone. Opioid-induced miosis or "pinpoint pupils" are mediated by increased muscarinic tone in the pupilloconstrictor neurons in the Edinger-Westphal nucleus,"[72] but this effect can be cloudy by hypoxic brain injury, concomitant drug use, or in opioids that have less miotic effects (meperidine, propoxyphene). Seizure after opioid overdose is uncommon but should be considered after prolonged downtime or if a pro-convulsant opioid (tramadol, meperidine, propoxyphene) was used.

The withdrawal syndrome of opioids is well-defined and characterized by objective (tachycardia, hypertension, piloerection, diarrhea, yawning) and subjective (irritability, anxiety, dysphoria, diminished motivation, malaise, abdominal cramping, muscle aches) signs and symptoms after the abrupt cessation of an opioid in a physically dependent person. Onset of symptoms is variable and depends on the pharmacokinetics, timing of last use, and chronicity of use prior to cessation. Although opioid withdrawal is uncomfortable, it is generally not life threatening. The degree of physical dependence does not predict the severity of craving. Drug craving may be protracted and result from the reduction of dopamine release in the nucleus accumbens. Protracted withdrawal is hypothesized to extend for an additional 1 to 4 weeks following the resolution of the acute withdrawal syndrome.[73]

Long-term opioid use induces tolerance to analgesic effects, physical and psychological dependence, opioid-induced hyperalgesia, and addiction. Many patients start using opioids for euphoria or for pain control. However, over time, increased doses are needed to provide the same relief and to avoid withdrawal or cravings, leading to a longer course than initially planned. After repeated expose to opioids, the brain undergoes complex neurobiological adaptations in the mesolimbic and locus ceruleus.[74] The mesolimbic system is responsible for most drug-associated reward and plays a role in the affective signs and symptoms of protracted opioid withdrawal. In contrast, physical dependence and somatic opioid withdrawal complaints that occur with acute withdrawal are primarily due to alterations in the locus ceruleus and noradrenergic system. Physical dependence to opioids varies in individuals (eg, genetic predisposition to opioid addiction), but can develop quickly and the neurobiological changes associated with regular use can escalate into OUD.[75]

Opioid receptor activation can lead to phosphorylation by many G-protein receptor kinases, and through complex cellular processes, the MOP will be degraded or recycled back to the cell membrane.[76] This decrease in MOP expression may contribute to tolerance and heighten sensitivity to pain leading to opioid-induced hyperalgesia.[74]

After an acute opioid overdose, providers should be cognizant of patients who receive naloxone and should carefully monitor for recurrence of symptoms. The half-life of opioids vary and may be active longer than the naloxone (half-life 30–60 minutes). If patients choose to leave the ED, they should be counseled on the risk of repeat respiratory depression, altered level of consciousness, and death. All patients that present for acute opioid withdrawal or opioid withdrawal should be counseled on harm reduction strategies, overdose education, offered naloxone, and medication to treat opioid use disorder, including buprenorphine or naltrexone.[77]

In addition to the effects of acute overdose, patients are at high risk of other complications resulting from the injection of contaminated adulterants (eg, quinine, talc) or infectious diseases like viral hepatitis, human immunodeficiency virus (HIV), sepsis, or endocarditis. This can lead to a complicated and prolonged hospital course; at which time the patient will also be experiencing opioid withdrawal and cravings and are at high risk of leaving prior to the completion of therapy. Patients with opioid use disorder should be offered treatment with medications for OUD (MOUD) like methadone or buprenorphine, as well as engagement in cognitive behavioral therapy or contingency management programs. Although MOUD can decrease the incidence of opioid overdose, addiction, and death, access to comfortable and appropriate providers is limited and existing legal barriers to prescribing make it a less appealing alternative to many providers. Other medications are described in the treatment of OUD in conjunction with MOUD to treat additional symptomatology (eg, clonidine to modulate symptoms via locus coeruleus–mediated noradrenergic hyperactivity).[73]

Nicotine

Nicotine is the principal alkaloid derived from the tobacco plant (genus *Nicotiana, family Solanaceae*). However, the primary human use and exposure is by use of cigarettes, cigars, other tobacco products. Nicotine is well-absorbed through multiple routes of exposure including the respiratory tract, mucosal surfaces, mucous membranes, and in the gastrointestinal tract. Depending on the route, nicotine is absorbed by the body at different rates but is generally rapidly absorbed. Distribution to body tissues is rapid and extensive. However, metabolism varies by the individual (race, gender, genetic polymorphism) leading to varying peak plasma concentrations.[78–80]

Nicotine binds the nicotinic cholinergic receptor, a ligand-gated ion channel receptor. Various nicotinic acetylcholine receptors have been identified and are involved in nicotine addiction. The $\alpha4\beta2^*$ nicotinic acetylcholine receptor has been identified as the most involved. This receptor is located on dopamine neurons, neurons projecting onto the DA neurons' cell bodies, and gamma-aminobutyric acid (GABA) and glutamate neurons. This allows nicotine to stimulate dopamine neurons by multiple mechanisms[1]: direct action on the $\alpha4\beta2^*$ nicotinic acetylcholine receptors on dopamine neurons, producing a brief response,[2] desensitization by nicotine on the receptors can cause an increase of glutamate to GABA transmission in the midbrain resulting in sustained activation of dopamine neurons, specifically the mesocorticolimbic system leading to the initial rewarding and reinforcing effects of nicotine.[81]

The mechanism of action and desired clinical effects of nicotine are dose dependent. Low doses of nicotine stimulate nicotinic receptors centrally and autonomic and somatic motor nerve fibers, classically producing increased mydriasis, heart rate, respiratory rate, blood pressure, and level of alertness. Onset of signs and symptoms are dependent on route of exposure. Early phase findings occur within 15 minutes to 1 hour. The duration of symptoms is about 1 to 2 hours following mild exposure.[82]

The intoxication syndrome of nicotine results from excessive nicotinic stimulation and receptor blockade with parasympathetic and neuromuscular-blocking effects, leading to vomiting, muscle fasciculations seizures, and dysrhythmias, bradycardia, hypotension, respiratory muscle weakness or paralysis, and death. These can occur within 30 minutes to 4 hours. The duration of symptoms is up to 18 to 24 hours following severe exposure. Death may occur within 1 hour after severe exposure. High-concentration electronic cigarette cartridges can cause severe intoxication and death when children accidently consume the contents.[83] There is no specific antidote for nicotine toxicity. Treatment of acute nicotine toxicity is symptomatic and supportive care, with a priority on airway protection and respiratory support.

Nicotine acts on the nicotine receptor, but also stimulates glutaminergic activation and the GABA (γ-aminobutyric acid)-ergic inhibition of dopaminergic neurons in the hippocampus, basal forebrain, and ventral tegmental area of the midbrain. These pathways are key neuromodulatory pathways for drug-induced reward, dependence, and withdrawal. The behavioral responses of pleasure and reward from nicotine use mainly results from dopamine, but also involves the actions of norepinephrine, acetylcholine, GABA, serotonin, glutamate, and endorphins. When exposed to nicotine, all the neurotransmitters are released and result in cognitive and mood improvement, appetite suppression, increased basal energy expenditures, and anxiety reduction. The rate of metabolism of nicotine is at least in part related to its addictive potential, with fast metabolizers having a higher rate of dependence and more difficultly quitting, while slow metabolizers smoke less, are less likely to be dependent, and have an easier time quitting.[84]

The nicotine withdrawal state begins after a drop in serum nicotine levels and is also associated with decreased levels of dopamine in the brain. Nicotine withdrawal syndromes are associated with a decrease of dopamine levels in the nucleus accumbens.[85] Nicotine withdrawal symptoms generally peak during the first 72 hours and then gradually subside over a 3–to-4-week period.[86] These symptoms can include restlessness, anxiety, difficulty concentrating, irritability, frustration, depression, and craving for cigarettes. Nicotine exposure is associated with tobacco exposure but are not mutually exclusive. While long-term cigarette use is associated with increased rates of chronic obstructive pulmonary disease (COPD), cardiovascular disease, pulmonary infections, macular degeneration, and cancers, chronic nicotine exposure causes cardiovascular damage related to catecholamine release and vasoconstriction.[87] Additionally, the separation of nicotine habituation and addiction is a difficult distinction as smoking a cigarette is more complex than a physical dependence on nicotine addiction. Food and Drug Administration-approved pharmacologic options for the treatment of tobacco use disorder include varenicline, bupropion and nicotine replacement therapy. When possible, combination of behavioral support plus pharmacotherapy is superior compared with pharmacotherapy alone.[88]

Halogenated, and Non-halogenated, Hydrocarbons

Hydrocarbons are chemicals that primarily contain carbon and hydrogen atoms. They may be aliphatic (straight-chain) or aromatic (cyclic). Halogenated hydrocarbons are hydrocarbons that also contain halogen atoms in the structure (eg, fluorine, chlorine, or bromine). Both these chemical classes are ubiquitous in modern life. However, while hydrocarbons can range from gases at room temperature to thick oils, the volatile ones are more commonly abused for their euphoric effect. Additional factors, such as lipophilicity, viscosity, and surface tension also impact the toxicity. These are sold as solvents, degreasers, paint thinners, pressurized gas, and refrigerants, among other uses. While there are numerous compounds, each with somewhat specific toxicities, as a group, hydrocarbons, and halogenated hydrocarbons share some specific concerns that are generalizable across different compounds.

Abuse of hydrocarbons is typically in the form in inhalation. Ingestion is generally limited to mild gastrointestinal upset for most hydrocarbons, although there is a significant risk of aspiration pneumonitis from the disruption of surfactant, if vomiting occurs. The different methods people use to inhale these agents are sniffing (direct inhalation from a container), huffing (inhaling the chemical from a pre-soaked cloth while holding it over the nose and mouth), and bagging (breathing in vapor from a paper or plastic bag containing the substance). Owing to the high lipophilicity, the compounds are rapidly absorbed into the blood stream and readily cross the blood brain barrier. They are also known to cross the placenta of pregnant women and expose the fetus as well. They are also rapidly eliminated, primarily through respiration, and only cause a short duration of intoxication.

Hydrocarbons are anesthetics, however, the exact mechanism by which they cause CNS depression isn't fully known. At least some of the chemicals in this class are reversible NMDA receptor antagonists.[89] However, paradoxically, with chronic use, it appears there is enhanced NMDA activity.[90] The chemicals also appear to increase GABA-Ar and glycine (the major inhibitory neurotransmitter of the spine) receptor activity, although how this is performed is not known.

Hydrocarbons also appear to activate dopaminergic neurons in the mesolimbic system, which increases the dopamine concentrations in the caudate nucleus and nucleus accumbens in rats.[91] In self-administration studies, rodents, primates, and humans have all shown reinforcing behavior with the use of hydrocarbons. Tolerance can form with chronic and frequent use. Withdrawal can occur but is primarily mild withdrawal syndrome. There is cross-tolerance to ethanol, benzodiazepines, and barbiturates. In addition, there are a myriad of other receptors that hydrocarbons appear to affect, including serotonin, nicotinic, and acetylcholine receptors. The effects from these other receptors are dose and substance dependent.

Other than anesthesia, there are specific toxicities associated with the use of certain hydrocarbons. Some hydrocarbons, such as n-hexane and methyl n-butyl ketone, are metabolized by the liver and cause peripheral neuropathy. Methylene chloride is metabolized to carbon monoxide and can rise to significant and dangerous levels. Halogenated hydrocarbons are known to induce arrythmias from the sensitization of the myocardium to epinephrine. The typical presentation is a patient who is started while sniffing who goes into cardiac arrest, termed "sudden sniffing death." Epinephrine should not be used in this scenario, as it can worsen the arrhythmia, and instead a betablocker such as esmolol is preferred. Halogenated hydrocarbons also cause negative inotropy, negative dromotropy, and negative chronotropy.[92] Chronic use of toluene can result in a non-anion gap metabolic acidosis associated with hypokalemia and hyperchloremia from a distal renal tubular acidosis. Lastly, as all hydrocarbons can serve as lipophilic solvents, they are associated with the defatting of the tissue they contact, as well as progressive encephalopathy from demyelination.

While some of these complications may be reversible, if use is significant enough, these pathologies can be permanent. A good history and observant physical examination for subtle signs of defatting, freezer burn or cold injuries from sniffing compressed gas, or evidence of metallic paint on the face (metallic spray paint has a higher concentration of toluene than non-metallic paint) can help identify patients at risk and help connect them to care to treat their use disorder. There is no specific antidote or treatment for hydrocarbon exposure, except the cessation of use.

Nitrous Oxide

Nitrous oxide (N_2O) is a colorless, nonirritant gas. It can induce euphoria, anxiolysis, and hallucinations. Its anesthetic properties result from NMDA antagonism, and the analgesic properties from endogenous opioid release in the midbrain which modulates pain processing in the spinal cord.[93] Due to the pleasurable high it produces, the term "laughing gas" was coined. Medicinally, it is used as an inhaled anesthetic owing to its analgesic and anxiolytic effects and is widely used in dentistry as well as during labor. It is also used in industry as a propellant and foaming agent for whipped cream, which is where it gets its street name "whippets."

Nitrous oxide abuse has been increasing, likely due to the fact it is a legal chemical and easy to obtain, owing to its use as a propellant and foaming agent for cream, and its perceived safety in comparison to other street drugs.[94] It is typically used by the inhalation of the gas from a balloon, which allows for the inhalation of near 100% nitrous oxide. It is rapidly absorbed, producing the desired effects within seconds. Peak effect is felt in about a minute, which completely disappears after a few minutes without a hangover or withdrawal effect. While a single hit carries little risk, repeated use and chronic use does carry significant long-term risks.

An example of how easy it is to obtain this drug is that on www.amazon.com you can purchase 600 whipped cream charger cartridges for only $177.09. Additionally, below the initial description, amazon recommends 2 additional purchases, that are frequently purchased together; a whipped cream dispense and 30 punch balloons, which are used to take a "hit" of nitrous oxide. One of the comments that gave 5-stars mentioned that the containers "work for what I got them for, and they also make whipped cream. Great price. Happy to have got them in bulk."[95]

Nitrous oxide is highly water soluble, allowing for rapid absorption across the alveolar membrane. This also ultimately leads to hypoxia from decreased oxygen absorption, which is typically short-lived and well-tolerated by a healthy individual, particularly in a well-ventilated space. However, in people with an underlying seizure disorder or cardiac disease, seizure, arrhythmias, and cardiac arrest have been documented.[96] Long-term consequences arise through a functional vitamin B12 (cobalamin) deficiency and primarily manifest as myelopathy and peripheral neuropathy, but can include delusions, delirium, and depression.

Nitrous oxide irreversibly oxidizes the cobalt ion in cobalamin, from the active 1+ state to 3+ and 2+ valence states, both of which are inactive. Vitamin B12 has 2 active forms, methylcobalamin and adenosylcobalamin. Methylcobalamin is a cofactor of methionine synthase (MTR), an enzyme that converts 5-methyltetrahydrofolate and homocysteine to tetrahydrofolate and methionine, and ultimately S-adenosylmethionine. A deficiency of this leads to a decrease of methionine and S-adenosylmethionine, which affects the methylation of myeline phospholipids, leading to the demyelination of the brain, spinal cord, and peripheral nervous system, megaloblastic anemia, and even optic nerve atrophy.[97] Additionally, the inability to metabolize homocysteine leads to toxic levels through oxidative stress through reactive oxygen species and NMDA mediated apoptosis.

Clinically, patients most commonly will present with symptoms of subacute combined degeneration (SCD) which is the demyelination of the posterior and lateral columns in the spinal cord, demyelination of white matter in the brain, and peripheral neuropathy.[98] These include paresthesia, decreased proprioception and vibration, weakness, and spasticity. Sensory deficits typically affect the longest nerves first, starting with the feet, and thn eventually the hands, and is associated with varying degrees of ataxia. These symptoms are more typical in long-term and severe use, however, patients with preexisting vitamin B12 deficiency are prone to developing symptoms sooner.

Nitrous oxide is not known to cause physical addiction, but regular use can lead to a psychological dependence. Treatment for patients with neurologic symptoms is primarily cessation of use to prevent further neurologic damage and vitamin B12 supplementation. However, there is no standard replacement protocol that is universally accepted. Most symptoms will improve or resolve; some patients may have permanent neurologic damage. Continued use of nitrous oxide is a poor prognostic indicator.

SUMMARY

There are numerous substances that are used recreationally and that have addictive potential. Each substance type carries unique and concerning risks, however, substance users frequently use multiple substances at once, creating a complex and often confusing clinical picture. Taking the time to obtain a full history and detailed physical exam can help to identify key aspects in each patient that can help clue in the clinician as to what substances may have been used and the end-organ effects that may be present.

CLINICS CARE POINTS

- Substance use and mental health disorders can be intricately related, and both must be addressed to best help the patient with a use disorder.

- Prompt recognition of drug toxidromes will help to identify the immediate toxicologic concerns and help guide long-term management options for substance use disorders.
- Most overdoses do not require the use of an antidote and the patients will recover with supportive care. For opioid overdoses with respiratory depression, the antidote of choice is naloxone.
- Sedative hypnotic withdrawal, which include ethanol withdrawal, can be deadly and requires careful consideration for medically managed detoxification.
- Substance use disorders are not the fault of the afflicted patients, but a true disease process that requires compassion and a firm understanding of the neurobiochemical causes to be able to properly address the causes and barriers to treatment and management our patients require.

DISCLOSURE

The authors have nothing to disclose. The views and opinions expressed in this article/ presentation are those of the author(s) and do not necessarily reflect official policy or position of the United States Air Force, Defense Health Agency, Department of Defense, or U.S. Government.

REFERENCES

1. CDC: National Center for Health Statistics. U.S. Overdose Deaths In 2021 Increased Half as Much as in 2020 – But Are Still Up 15% 2022 Available at: https://www.cdc.gov/nchs/pressroom/nchs_press_releases/2022/202205.htm.   Accessed December 15, 2022.
2. Peterson C, Li M, Xu L, et al. Assessment of Annual Cost of Substance Use Disorder in US Hospitals. JAMA Netw Open 2021;4(3):e210242.
3. Jones CM, McCance-Katz EF. Co-occurring substance use and mental disorders among adults with opioid use disorder. Drug Alcohol Depend 2019;197:78–82.
4. U.S. Department of Health &Human Services. Substance abuse and mental health Services administration. The National Survey on Drug Use and Health; 2022.
5. Curry A. A 9,000-year love affair. National Geographic; 2017.
6. Li F, Tsien JZ. Memory and the NMDA receptors. N Engl J Med 2009;361(3): 302–3.
7. Holland MG, Ferner RE. A systematic review of the evidence for acute tolerance to alcohol - the "Mellanby effect". Clin Toxicol 2017;55(6):545–56.
8. Gaw CE, Osterhoudt KC. Ethanol Intoxication of Young Children. Pediatr Emerg Care 2019;35(10):722–30.
9. Koob GF, Colrain IM. Alcohol use disorder and sleep disturbances: a feed-forward allostatic framework. Neuropsychopharmacology 2020;45(1):141–65.
10. Wijnia JW. A Clinician's View of Wernicke-Korsakoff Syndrome. J Clin Med 2022; 11(22):6755.
11. Singh S, Wagh V. Marchiafava Bignami Disease: A Rare Neurological Complication of Long-Term Alcohol Abuse. Cureus 2022;14(10):e30863.
12. Day E, Rudd JHF. Alcohol use disorders and the heart. Addiction 2019;114(9): 1670–8.
13. Voskoboinik A, McDonald C, Chieng D, et al. Acute electrical, autonomic and structural effects of binge drinking: Insights into the 'holiday heart syndrome'. Int J Cardiol 2021;331:100–5.

14. Sanghvi SR, Kellerman PS, Nanovic L. Beer potomania: an unusual cause of hyponatremia at high risk of complications from rapid correction. Am J Kidney Dis 2007;50(4):673–80.

15. Lodhi MU, Saleem TS, Kuzel AR, et al. "Beer Potomania" - A Syndrome of Severe Hyponatremia with Unique Pathophysiology: Case Studies and Literature Review. Cureus 2017;9(12):e2000.

16. National Institute on Alcohol Abuse and Alcooholism. Drinking Levels Defined Available from: https://www.niaaa.nih.gov/alcohol-health/overview-alcohol-consumption/moderate-binge-drinking. Accessed December 15, 2022.

17. Addolorato G, Vassallo GA, Antonelli G, et al. Binge Drinking among adolescents is related to the development of Alcohol Use Disorders: results from a Cross-Sectional Study. Sci Rep 2018;8(1):12624.

18. Nieto SJ, Baskerville W, Donato S, et al. Lifetime heavy drinking years predict alcohol use disorder severity over and above current alcohol use. Am J Drug Alcohol Abuse 2021;47(5):630–7.

19. Jesse S, Brathen G, Ferrara M, et al. Alcohol withdrawal syndrome: mechanisms, manifestations, and management. Acta Neurol Scand 2017;135(1):4–16.

20. Castillo-Carniglia A, Keyes KM, Hasin DS, et al. Psychiatric comorbidities in alcohol use disorder. Lancet Psychiatr 2019;6(12):1068–80.

21. McHugh RK, Weiss RD. Alcohol Use Disorder and Depressive Disorders. Alcohol Res 2019;40(1):e1–8. https://doi.org/10.35946/arcr.v40.1.01. PMID: 31649834.

22. Nunes EV, Liu X, Samet S, et al. Independent versus substance-induced major depressive disorder in substance-dependent patients: observational study of course during follow-up. J Clin Psychiatry 2006;67(10):1561–7.

23. Amiri S, Behnezhad S. Alcohol use and risk of suicide: a systematic review and Meta-analysis. J Addict Dis 2020;38(2):200–13.

24. Edwards AC, Ohlsson H, Sundquist J, et al. Alcohol Use Disorder and Risk of Suicide in a Swedish Population-Based Cohort. Am J Psychiatry 2020;177(7):627–34.

25. U.S. Department of Health and Human Services: Substance Abuse and Mental Health Services Administration. Key Substance Use and Mental Health Indicators in the United States: Results from the 2019 National Survey on Drug Use and Health Available from: https://www.samhsa.gov/data/sites/default/files/reports/rpt29393/2019NSDUHFFRPDFWHTML/2019NSDUHFFR090120.htm. Accessed December 15, 2022.

26. Esser MB, Sherk A, Liu Y, et al. Deaths and Years of Potential Life Lost From Excessive Alcohol Use - United States, 2011-2015. MMWR Morb Mortal Wkly Rep 2020;69(39):1428–33.

27. Derry JM, Dunn SM, Davies M. Identification of a residue in the gamma-aminobutyric acid type A receptor alpha subunit that differentially affects diazepam-sensitive and -insensitive benzodiazepine site binding. J Neurochem 2004;88(6):1431–8.

28. Vinkers CH, Olivier B. Mechanisms Underlying Tolerance after Long-Term Benzodiazepine Use: A Future for Subtype-Selective GABA(A) Receptor Modulators? Adv Pharmacol Sci 2012;2012:416864.

29. Touitou Y. [Sleep disorders and hypnotic agents: medical, social and economical impact]. Ann Pharm Fr 2007;65(4):230–8.

30. Huedo-Medina TB, Kirsch I, Middlemass J, et al. Effectiveness of non-benzodiazepine hypnotics in treatment of adult insomnia: meta-analysis of data submitted to the Food and Drug Administration. BMJ 2012;345:e8343.

31. Siriwardena AN, Qureshi MZ, Dyas JV, et al. Magic bullets for insomnia? Patients' use and experiences of newer (Z drugs) versus older (benzodiazepine) hypnotics for sleep problems in primary care. Br J Gen Pract 2008;58(551):417–22.

32. Edinoff AN, Nix CA, Hollier J, et al. Benzodiazepines: Uses, Dangers, and Clinical Considerations. Neurol Int 2021;13(4):594–607.

33. Tan KR, Rudolph U, Luscher C. Hooked on benzodiazepines: GABAA receptor subtypes and addiction. Trends Neurosci 2011;34(4):188–97.

34. Gueye PN, Hoffman JR, Taboulet P, et al. Empiric use of flumazenil in comatose patients: limited applicability of criteria to define low risk. Ann Emerg Med 1996;27(6):730–5.

35. Kreshak AA, Cantrell FL, Clark RF, et al. A poison center's ten-year experience with flumazenil administration to acutely poisoned adults. J Emerg Med 2012;43(4):677–82.

36. Nguyen TT, Troendle M, Cumpston K, et al. Lack of adverse effects from flumazenil administration: an ED observational study. Am J Emerg Med 2015;33(11):1677–9.

37. Chudnofsky CR. Safety and efficacy of flumazenil in reversing conscious sedation in the emergency department. Emergency Medicine Conscious Sedation Study Group. Acad Emerg Med 1997;4(10):944–50.

38. Hood SD, Norman A, Hince DA, et al. Benzodiazepine dependence and its treatment with low dose flumazenil. Br J Clin Pharmacol 2014;77(2):285–94.

39. Adinoff B. Neurobiologic processes in drug reward and addiction. Harv Rev Psychiatry 2004;12(6):305–20.

40. Daras M, Koppel BS, Atos-Radzion E. Cocaine-induced choreoathetoid movements ('crack dancing'). Neurology 1994;44(4):751–2.

41. Isenschmid D. Cocaine. In: Levine BS, Kerrigan S, editors. Principles of forensic toxicology. Cham: Springer; 2020.

42. Lange RA, Hillis LD. Cardiovascular complications of cocaine use. N Engl J Med 2001;345(5):351–8.

43. Bauman JL, DiDomenico RJ. Cocaine-induced channelopathies: emerging evidence on the multiple mechanisms of sudden death. J Cardiovasc Pharmacol Ther 2002;7(3):195–202.

44. Forrester JM, Steele AW, Waldron JA, et al. Crack lung: an acute pulmonary syndrome with a spectrum of clinical and histopathologic findings. Am Rev Respir Dis 1990;142(2):462–7.

45. Harris DS, Everhart ET, Mendelson J, et al. The pharmacology of cocaethylene in humans following cocaine and ethanol administration. Drug Alcohol Depend 2003;72(2):169–82.

46. Kirby LG, Zeeb FD, Winstanley CA. Contributions of serotonin in addiction vulnerability. Neuropharmacology 2011;61(3):421–32.

47. American College of Emergency Physicians Hyperactive Delirium Task Force. ACEP Task Force Report on Hyperactive Delirium with Severe Agitation in Emergency Settings. 2021 6/23/2021.

48. Mustaquim D, Jones CM, Compton WM. Trends and correlates of cocaine use among adults in the United States, 2006-2019. Addict Behav 2021;120:106950.

49. Rounsaville BJ. Treatment of cocaine dependence and depression. Biol Psychiatry 2004;56(10):803–9.

50. Singh VM, Browne T, Montgomery J. The Emerging Role of Toxic Adulterants in Street Drugs in the US Illicit Opioid Crisis. Public Health Rep 2020;135(1):6–10.

51. Bentzley BS, Han SS, Neuner S, et al. Comparison of Treatments for Cocaine Use Disorder Among Adults: A Systematic Review and Meta-analysis. JAMA Netw Open 2021;4(5):e218049.
52. Seiden LS, Kleven MS. Methamphetamine and related drugs: toxicity and resulting behavioral changes in response to pharmacological probes. NIDA Res Monogr 1989;94:146–60.
53. Hirata H, Ladenheim B, Rothman RB, et al. Methamphetamine-induced serotonin neurotoxicity is mediated by superoxide radicals. Brain Res 1995;677(2):345–7.
54. Baumann MH, Ayestas MA, Sharpe LG, et al. Persistent antagonism of methamphetamine-induced dopamine release in rats pretreated with GBR12909 decanoate. J Pharmacol Exp Ther 2002;301(3):1190–7.
55. Sellers EM, Otton SV, Tyndale RF. The potential role of the cytochrome P-450 2D6 pharmacogenetic polymorphism in drug abuse. NIDA Res Monogr 1997; 173:6–26.
56. McCutcheon RA, Krystal JH, Howes OD. Dopamine and glutamate in schizophrenia: biology, symptoms and treatment. World Psychiatr 2020;19(1):15–33.
57. Sara GE, Large MM, Matheson SL, et al. Stimulant use disorders in people with psychosis: a meta-analysis of rate and factors affecting variation. Aust N Z J Psychiatry 2015;49(2):106–17.
58. Shoptaw SJ, Kao U, Ling WW. Treatment for amphetamine psychosis. Cochrane Database Syst Rev 2008;4:CD003026.
59. The Health Effects of Cannabis and Cannabinoids. The current state of evidence and Recommendations for Research. Washington (DC): The National Academies Collection: Reports funded by National Institutes of Health; 2017.
60. Bloomfield MA, Ashok AH, Volkow ND, et al. The effects of Delta(9)-tetrahydrocannabinol on the dopamine system. Nature 2016;539(7629):369–77.
61. Howlett AC, Abood ME. CB(1) and CB(2) Receptor Pharmacology. Adv Pharmacol 2017;80:169–206.
62. Madras BK. Tinkering with THC-to-CBD ratios in Marijuana. Neuropsychopharmacology 2019;44(1):215–6.
63. Potts AJ, Cano C, Thomas SHL, et al. Synthetic cannabinoid receptor agonists: classification and nomenclature. Clin Toxicol (Phila) 2020;58(2):82–98.
64. Tait RJ, Caldicott D, Mountain D, et al. A systematic review of adverse events arising from the use of synthetic cannabinoids and their associated treatment. Clin Toxicol 2016;54(1):1–13.
65. Desrosiers NA, Ramaekers JG, Chauchard E, et al. Smoked cannabis' psychomotor and neurocognitive effects in occasional and frequent smokers. J Anal Toxicol 2015;39(4):251–61.
66. American Psychiatric Association. Diagnostic and statistical manual of mental disorders : DSM-5-TR. In: Text revision. 5th edition. Washington, DC: American Psychiatric Association Publishing; 2022. p. 1050.
67. Bahji A, Stephenson C, Tyo R, et al. Prevalence of Cannabis Withdrawal Symptoms Among People With Regular or Dependent Use of Cannabinoids: A Systematic Review and Meta-analysis. JAMA Netw Open 2020;3(4):e202370.
68. Lac A, Luk JW. Testing the Amotivational Syndrome: Marijuana Use Longitudinally Predicts Lower Self-Efficacy Even After Controlling for Demographics, Personality, and Alcohol and Cigarette Use. Prev Sci 2018;19(2):117–26.
69. Stein C. Opioid Receptors. Annu Rev Med 2016;67:433–51.
70. Hemby SE, Martin TJ, Co C, et al. The effects of intravenous heroin administration on extracellular nucleus accumbens dopamine concentrations as determined by in vivo microdialysis. J Pharmacol Exp Ther 1995;273(2):591–8.

71. Aicher SA, Goldberg A, Sharma S. Co-localization of mu opioid receptor and N-methyl-D-aspartate receptor in the trigeminal dorsal horn. J Pain 2002;3(3): 203–10.

72. Rollins MD, Feiner JR, Lee JM, et al. Pupillary effects of high-dose opioid quantified with infrared pupillometry. Anesthesiology 2014;121(5):1037–44.

73. Dunn KE, Huhn AS, Bergeria CL, et al. Non-Opioid Neurotransmitter Systems that Contribute to the Opioid Withdrawal Syndrome: A Review of Preclinical and Human Evidence. J Pharmacol Exp Ther 2019;371(2):422–52.

74. Colvin LA, Bull F, Hales TG. Perioperative opioid analgesia-when is enough too much? A review of opioid-induced tolerance and hyperalgesia. Lancet 2019; 393(10180):1558–68.

75. Eippert F, Bingel U, Schoell ED, et al. Activation of the opioidergic descending pain control system underlies placebo analgesia. Neuron 2009;63(4):533–43.

76. Zhang L, Kibaly C, Wang YJ, et al. Src-dependent phosphorylation of mu-opioid receptor at Tyr(336) modulates opiate withdrawal. EMBO Mol Med 2017;9(11): 1521–36.

77. Hawk K, Hoppe J, Ketcham E, et al. Consensus Recommendations on the Treatment of Opioid Use Disorder in the Emergency Department. Ann Emerg Med 2021;78(3):434–42.

78. Benowitz NL, Lessov-Schlaggar CN, Swan GE, et al. Female sex and oral contraceptive use accelerate nicotine metabolism. Clin Pharmacol Ther 2006;79(5): 480–8.

79. Perez-Stable EJ, Herrera B, Jacob P 3rd, et al. Nicotine metabolism and intake in black and white smokers. JAMA 1998;280(2):152–6.

80. Malaiyandi V, Sellers EM, Tyndale RF. Implications of CYP2A6 genetic variation for smoking behaviors and nicotine dependence. Clin Pharmacol Ther 2005;77(3): 145–58.

81. Bozinoff N, Le Foll B. Understanding the implications of the biobehavioral basis of nicotine addiction and its impact on the efficacy of treatment. Expert Rev Respir Med 2018;12(9):793–804.

82. The National Institute for Occupational Safety and Health. Nicotine: Systemic Agent Available at: https://www.cdc.gov/niosh/ershdb/emergencyresponsecard_ 29750028.html. Accessed December 15, 2022.

83. McGrath-Morrow SA, Gorzkowski J, Groner JA, et al. The Effects of Nicotine on Development. Pediatrics 2020;145(3):e20191346.

84. Ray R, Tyndale RF, Lerman C. Nicotine dependence pharmacogenetics: role of genetic variation in nicotine-metabolizing enzymes. J Neurogenet 2009;23(3): 252–61.

85. Epping-Jordan MP, Watkins SS, Koob GF, et al. Dramatic decreases in brain reward function during nicotine withdrawal. Nature 1998;393(6680):76–9.

86. Martin-Soelch C. Neuroadaptive changes associated with smoking: structural and functional neural changes in nicotine dependence. Brain Sci 2013;3(1): 159–76.

87. Prevention CfDCa. Available at: https://www.cdc.gov/niosh/ershdb/ emergencyresponsecard_29750028.html . Accessed December 15, 2022.

88. Stead LF, Perera R, Bullen C, et al. Nicotine replacement therapy for smoking cessation. Cochrane Database Syst Rev 2012;11:CD000146.

89. Cruz SL, Balster RL, Woodward JJ. Effects of volatile solvents on recombinant N-methyl-D-aspartate receptors expressed in Xenopus oocytes. Br J Pharmacol 2000;131(7):1303–8.

90. Bale AS, Tu Y, Carpenter-Hyland EP, et al. Alterations in glutamatergic and ga-baergic ion channel activity in hippocampal neurons following exposure to the abused inhalant toluene. Neuroscience 2005;130(1):197–206.

91. Tormoehlen LM, Tekulve KJ, Nanagas KA. Hydrocarbon toxicity: A review. Clin Toxicol 2014;52(5):479–89.

92. Muller SP, Wolna P, Wunscher U, et al. Cardiotoxicity of chlorodibromomethane and trichloromethane in rats and isolated rat cardiac myocytes. Arch Toxicol 1997;71(12):766–77.

93. Temple C, Horowitz BZ. Nitrous oxide abuse induced subacute combined degen-eration despite patient initiated B12 supplementation. Clin Toxicol 2022;60(7): 872–5.

94. Kaar SJ, Ferris J, Waldron J, et al. Up: The rise of nitrous oxide abuse. An inter-national survey of contemporary nitrous oxide use. J Psychopharmacol 2016; 30(4):395–401.

95. Amazon product description for whipped cream cartidges Available at: https://www.amazon.com/dp/B09M8ZTTLZ/ref=redir_mobile_desktop?_encoding=UTF8&aaxitk=b0f8421ba8c040a8e144dcf0e84332b4&content-id=amzn1.sym.552bcbb2-81a1-4e8b-b868-3fba7d5af42a%3Aamzn1.sym.552bcbb2-81a1-4e8b-b868-3fba7d5af42a&hsa_cr_id=8277075060801&pd_rd_plhdr=t&pd_rd_r=2de01096-8eb4-4759-b3ca-dbdcb370104c&pd_rd_w=aTemM&pd_rd_wg=RElv2&qid=1670171568&ref_=sbx_be_s_sparkle_mcd_asin_0_title&sr=1-1-9e67e56a-6f64-441f-a281-df67fc737124. Accessed December 15, 2022.

96. Wagner SA, Clark MA, Wesche DL, et al. Asphyxial deaths from the recreational use of nitrous oxide. J Forensic Sci 1992;37(4):1008–15.

97. Xiang Y, Li L, Ma X, et al. Recreational Nitrous Oxide Abuse: Prevalence, Neuro-toxicity, and Treatment. Neurotox Res 2021;39(3):975–85.

98. Nouri A, Patel K, Montejo J, et al. The Role of Vitamin B(12) in the Management and Optimization of Treatment in Patients With Degenerative Cervical Myelopathy. Global Spine J 2019;9(3):331–7.

Schizophrenia and Emergency Medicine

Ryan E. Lawrence, MD[a],*, Adam Bernstein, MD[b]

KEYWORDS

- Schizophrenia • Schizoaffective disorder • Psychosis • Hallucinations • Delusions
- Agitation • Antipsychotic medication • Medical comorbidity

KEY POINTS

- Schizophrenia is a syndrome that can include a variety of symptoms, especially positive symptoms (hallucinations, delusions), negative symptoms (avolition, anhedonia, reduced social engagement), and disorganized thoughts and behaviors.
- Persons with schizophrenia may present to emergency departments for reasons directly related to schizophrenia as well as because of other mental health or medical problems.
- Antipsychotic medication (antagonists of the D2 dopamine receptor) has been a mainstay of treatment for decades, but persons also benefit from psychotherapy and supportive services.
- Persons with schizophrenia should be assessed for risk of suicide, risk of violence, risk of being unable to care for themselves, and risk of being the victims of violence as well as for other mental health and medical problems.

INTRODUCTION: EPIDEMIOLOGY

Schizophrenia and other psychotic disorders are commonly encountered around the world, with an estimated lifetime prevalence of 0.7%.[1] This number may seem small on a percentage basis, but it translates into an extremely large number of affected persons.

Persons with schizophrenia are also commonly encountered in emergency department (ED) settings. In part, this is because EDs have become important locations for persons with mental health problems to access care, likely due to many factors including being open 24 hours per day, providing evaluation and treatment regardless of an individual's ability to pay, and because community resources can be difficult to access.[2]

[a] Comprehensive Psychiatric Emergency Program, Columbia University Irving Medical Center and New York-Presbyterian Hospital, 622 West 168 Street, New York, NY 10032, USA; [b] Creedmoor Psychiatric Center, New York State Office of Mental Health, 79-25 Winchester Boulevard, Queens, NY 11427, USA
* Corresponding author.
E-mail address: rel2137@cumc.columbia.edu

Emerg Med Clin N Am 42 (2024) 93–104
https://doi.org/10.1016/j.emc.2023.06.012
0733-8627/24/© 2023 Elsevier Inc. All rights reserved.

emed.theclinics.com

Data from the United States National Center for Health Statistics indicate that adults with schizophrenia (operationalized in the study as persons with a diagnosis code 295 according to the International Classification of Diseases, Ninth Revision, Clinical Modification listed as a first, second, or third diagnosis) generate more than 380,000 ED visits per year, corresponding to an overall visit rate of 20.1 per 10,000 adults.[3] For a slight majority of these patients (58.8%), schizophrenia itself was the primary diagnosis and reason for the visit (eg, exacerbation of psychotic symptoms, agitation, disorganization, delusions, poor self-care). However, many persons with schizophrenia presented because of another mental health problem (15.4% had another mental disorder as the primary diagnosis), which might include depression, anxiety, or substance use. Persons also presented for reasons unrelated to their mental health (a nonmental health disorder was the primary diagnosis in 25.7% of visits), with complaints that included pain, acute injury, infectious processes, and a host of other medical concerns. Persons with schizophrenia presenting to EDs were especially likely to require medical hospitalization (32.7%) or psychiatric hospitalization (16.7%) in the study.

SCHIZOPHRENIA AS A DIAGNOSIS
Diagnostic Criteria

According to the Diagnostic and Statistical Manual of Mental Disorders, Fifth Edition, Text Revision (DSM-5-TR),[4] there are several core features seen across all psychotic disorders to varying degrees. These include delusions, hallucinations while fully awake, disorganized thinking, or speech that is severe enough to impair communication, disorganized or nonsensical behavior, and negative symptoms (avolition, diminished emotional expression, decreased speech output, anhedonia, and decreased engagement in social interaction). Culture and language must always be taken into account, as these shape expectations of what is considered normal versus abnormal.

For a diagnosis of schizophrenia to be rendered, symptoms must align with a specific time course and must include multiple domains (**Table 1**).[4] Importantly, as a heterogeneous clinical syndrome, there is no single symptom that is pathognomonic for the disorder.

Symptoms most commonly emerge in late adolescence or early adulthood, and the onset can be slow and gradual or abrupt and fulminant.[4] A prodromal period with attenuated symptoms may precede the active phase when symptoms are most prominent. Following an active phase, residual symptoms may remain. The long-term course can be highly variable, with some individuals experiencing severe, chronic, and refractory symptoms, whereas others experience periods of remission and even sustained recovery.

Associated Features

Several features are commonly associated with schizophrenia, even though they are not necessarily part of the diagnostic criteria.[4] Persons with schizophrenia may exhibit inappropriate affect, dysphoric or irritable mood (eg, depression, anxiety, anger), unusual sleep patterns (eg, day/night reversal), cognitive deficits (including problems with social cognition), reduced attention, and interpreting irrelevant events as somehow meaningful. Neurologic soft signs can be present, such as impaired motor coordination, left-right confusion, and disinhibition of associated movements. A lack of insight into one's symptoms is another commonly associated feature.

Table 1
Summary of diagnostic criteria for schizophrenia in the Diagnostic and Statistical Manual of Mental Disorders, Fifth Edition, Text Revision[4]

Criteria	Description
A	Symptoms in at least two areas must be present for a significant amount of time during a 1-mo period (can be shorter if a person is treated) 1. Delusional beliefs 2. Hallucinations 3. Disorganized thought process or speech 4. Significantly disorganized or catatonic behavior 5. Negative symptoms
B	Functioning has significantly declined since the onset of symptoms (eg, work, relationships, grooming, self-care)
C	Symptoms must be present for at least 6 mo, with at least 1 mo of active-phase symptoms (from Criterion A)
D&E	Other disorders have been ruled out (eg, schizoaffective disorder, bipolar disorder, depression with psychotic features, substance or medication-induced psychosis, psychosis due to another medical condition)
F	When autism spectrum disorder or a childhood onset communication disorder is present, schizophrenia is diagnosed only if delusions or hallucinations are prominent and all other diagnostic criteria for schizophrenia are present for at least 1 mo.

Differential Diagnosis

Schizophrenia is just one of many psychotic disorders. When an individual presents with psychotic symptoms, a broad differential diagnosis should be considered.[4] The timing of symptoms, their relative severity across different domains, and the identification of contributing factors (eg, substance use) are important for the diagnosis. A family history may also be informative. Making a precise diagnosis is important for shaping treatment plans and advising on the prognosis. **Table 2** summarizes some important features of other psychotic disorders that should be considered when evaluating a person for possible schizophrenia.

Recommendations for Medical Evaluation

Schizophrenia is presently a clinical diagnosis, meaning that there are no definitive imaging, laboratory, or psychological tests that generate or confirm the diagnosis. Nevertheless, a thorough medical evaluation remains essential for navigating the differential diagnosis and excluding other causes of psychotic symptoms. **Box 1** describes a variety of tests that should be considered, depending on the information obtained during the history and physical.

PATHOPHYSIOLOGY

Although much studied, the pathophysiology underlying schizophrenia remains incompletely understood. Evidence has long suggested that there are multiple contributing factors and perhaps more than one pathophysiological process resulting in a final common pathway. However, because the mid-twentieth century discovery that blockade of the D2 dopamine receptors is associated with reduced psychotic symptoms (namely hallucinations, delusions, and disorganization) dopamine has been a primary focus of research.

Table 2
Differential diagnosis: other psychotic disorders that should be considered when evaluating a person for schizophrenia

Diagnosis	Distinguishing Features
Major depression or bipolar disorder with psychotic features	Delusions or hallucinations occur exclusively during a major depressive or manic episode. Although mood symptoms are common among persons with schizophrenia, mood episodes should be present for a minority of the time during active and residual phases.
Schizotypal personality disorder	Pervasive social and interpersonal deficits beginning by early adulthood, with odd beliefs that are below the threshold for diagnosing a psychotic disorder
Delusional disorder	A delusion lasting at least 1 mo with no other psychotic symptoms and well-preserved functioning
Brief psychotic disorder	Psychosis lasting more than 1 d but remitting by 1 mo
Schizophreniform disorder	Symptoms resemble schizophrenia but the duration is <6 mo and overall functioning is preserved
Schizoaffective disorder	A mood episode and active-phase symptoms of schizophrenia co-occur and were preceded or followed by at least 2 wk of delusions or hallucinations without prominent mood symptoms; mood symptoms must be present for >50% of the total duration of the active periods
Obsessive-compulsive disorder and body dysmorphic disorder	Preoccupations can be severe enough to be considered delusional but are distinguished from schizophrenia by prominent obsessions, compulsions, or body-focused repetitive behaviors
Post-traumatic stress disorder	Flashbacks and hypervigilance may resemble psychosis, but a traumatic event and reexperiencing symptoms must also be present
Postpartum psychosis	Psychotic symptoms in the context of recent childbirth
Substance-induced psychotic disorder	Recent substance use with symptoms lasting longer than would be expected from acute intoxication
Psychosis due to a medical condition	A general medical condition is identified as the primary cause of psychotic symptoms (eg, epilepsy, systemic lupus erythematosus, other autoimmune diseases, tumor, dementia, endocrine disorders)
Psychosis from toxic exposure	Recent exposure to a medication or other toxin that causes psychosis

Sources: DSM-5-TR,[4] Lieberman & First 2018.[5]

Brain imaging studies have found robust evidence for dysfunction of the dopamine system in schizophrenia.[6] For example, radioligand displacement studies have found that persons with schizophrenia show increased dopamine release in response to low-dose amphetamine, which correlates with transient worsening of psychotic

Box 1
Suggested medical and neurologic tests when evaluating for schizophrenia
Complete blood count
Comprehensive metabolic panel
Thyroid-stimulating hormone level
Drug screen
Ethanol level
Inflammatory markers
Syphilis testing
Medication levels
Electroencephalogram (EEG)[a]
Brain imaging[a]
[a]EEG and brain imaging are not necessarily performed on all patients but are indicated if there is clinical suspicion for a neurologic event or process that these tests could evaluate.
Source: Lieberman & First, 2018.[5]

symptoms. Persons with schizophrenia show increased baseline levels of synaptic dopamine in the striatum. Elevated striatal dopamine synthesis capacity has also been observed and may correlate with the severity of psychotic symptoms. Elevations in striatal dopamine seem to be limited to striatal projections, whereas mesocortical projections (especially to the dorsolateral prefrontal cortex) have reduced dopamine release compared with healthy controls. Although there is little controversy about dysregulation of dopamine pathways being a core feature of psychotic symptoms in schizophrenia, dysregulation of other neurotransmitters (especially glutamate and gamma-aminobutyric acid) has also been implicated in the disorder.[7]

Genetic studies have provided several insights into the origins of schizophrenia.[7] Schizophrenia's heritability is high, approximately 80%, but in most cases, it seems not to be associated with any one gene. Linkage studies have identified several genes with important roles in neurodevelopment to be implicated in schizophrenia (erb-B2 receptor tyrosine kinase 4 [ERBB4], dystrobrevin binding protein 1 [DTNBP1], neuregulin 1 [NGR-1], disrupted in schizophrenia 1 [DISC1], AKT serine/threonine kinase 1 [AKT1], regulator of G-protein signaling 4 [RGS-4], catechol-O-methyltransferase [COMT], vesicular monoamine transporter 2 [VMAT2], and cardiomyopathy associated 5 [CMYA5]). Structural variations or copy number variants have been identified as well, often disrupting genes involved in neurodevelopmental pathways related to synaptic development and function (neurexin 1 [NRXN1], amyloid beta precursor protein binding family A member 2 [APBA2], neureglin 1 [NRG1], contactin associated protein 2 [CNTNAP2]). These variations tend to be unique and rare in the general population but can confer significant risk of schizophrenia to the affected individuals. Genome-wide association studies have also found well over 100 single-nucleotide polymorphisms that are associated with schizophrenia (eg, major histocompatibility complex [MHC] region of chromosome 6, neurogranin [NRGN], transcription factor 4 [TCF4]). Many of these single-nucleotide polymorphisms are associated with central immune functions, the D2 dopamine receptor, glutamatergic neurotransmission, and synaptic plasticity. These various discoveries suggest that schizophrenia is a disorder with a multifactorial etiology, likely involving multiple genetic risk factors which can interact with environmental factors to cause a symptomatic state.

Some important environmental factors have been identified that confer increased the risk of developing schizophrenia. Examples include maternal malnutrition during gestation, low maternal folate levels during pregnancy, maternal exposure to infection during gestation, obstetric complications, advanced paternal age, and living in an urban environment.[8]

A particular environmental exposure that has been associated with schizophrenia and other psychotic disorders is the use of cannabis and related products.[9] Both observational and experimental studies have identified an association between cannabis use and the onset and persistence of psychotic disorders. The risk of psychosis increases with more cannabis exposure, use at an earlier age, and use of higher potency and synthetic products containing high levels of tetrahydrocannabinol relative to cannabidiol (cannabidiol may lessen the psychotogenic effects of tetrahydrocannabinol). Because this is a potentially modifiable risk factor, it presents a rare opportunity to alter the schizophrenia burden in the population through public health education.

TREATING SCHIZOPHRENIA

The American Psychiatric Association (APA) issued new practice guidelines in 2021 that provide evidence-based recommendations for both pharmacologic and non-pharmacological treatments for schizophrenia.[10]

Pharmacologic Treatments

The APA recommends treating patients with schizophrenia with antipsychotic medication (D2 antagonists), with ongoing monitoring of treatment effectiveness and adverse effects.[10] If symptoms improve, the same antipsychotic medication should be continued. No algorithm exists to determine which antipsychotic should be selected; rather the choice is guided by the patient's preferences, treatment history, recovery goals, and an element of trial and error. **Table 3** describes the side effect profiles of some commonly used antipsychotic medications and illustrates the diversity of side effects that patients and prescribers must weigh when selecting an antipsychotic medication.

Many of these adverse effects have effective treatments.[10] Acute dystonia should be treated with anticholinergic medication (eg, benztropine or diphenhydramine). Common practice is to change the antipsychotic medication if acute dystonia occurs. Parkinsonism can be treated by reducing the dose of the antipsychotic medication,

Table 3
Side effect profiles of some commonly used antipsychotic medications

| Medication | Level of Risk for Each Adverse Effect | | | | |
	Akathisia	Parkinsonism	Sedation	Dystonia	Weight Gain
Chlorpromazine	Moderate	Moderate	High	Moderate	Moderate
Haloperidol	High	High	Low	High	Low
Aripiprazole	Moderate	Low	Low	Low	Low
Clozapine	Low	Low	High	Low	High
Olanzapine	Moderate	Moderate	High	Low	High
Risperidone	Moderate	Moderate	Moderate	Moderate	Moderate

Adapted from APA 2021.[10]

changing to a different antipsychotic medication (eg, quetiapine), or treating with anti-cholinergic medication. If akathisia occurs (uncomfortable restlessness and urge to move), the antipsychotic medication dose can be lowered, the patient can switch to a different antipsychotic medication, a benzodiazepine can be added to the treatment regimen, or a beta-adrenergic blocking agent can be added. For patients who develop moderate to severe tardive dyskinesia (frequently taking the form of involuntary movements of facial muscles), a trial of a reversible inhibitor of the VMAT2 is indicated.

Among the antipsychotic medication options, clozapine is specifically recommended in a few circumstances: when patients have treatment-resistant symptoms, when there is a substantial risk of suicide, or when there is high risk for violence or agitation.[10] Unlike other antipsychotic medications, where the dose can be escalated rapidly once tolerability is established, clozapine requires a slow titration to minimize risks of seizure, excessive sedation, and orthostatic hypotension. In the United States, patients who receive clozapine must be registered with the Risk Evaluation and Mitigation Strategy program, which tracks the patient's absolute neutrophil count to avoid potentially life-threatening neutropenia.

Long-acting injectables exist for some antipsychotic medications and can be used for patients with poor or uncertain adherence or for patients who prefer this route of administration.[10] Commonly, an oral formulation is used first, in order to establish tolerability and effectiveness, and then the patient transitions to the long-acting injectable.

A rare but potentially fatal medical emergency that can occur in the context of antipsychotic treatment is neuroleptic malignant syndrome, which is identified by the triad of rigidity, hyperthermia, and sympathetic nervous system lability (including hypertension and tachycardia).[10] Additional features often include elevated serum creatine kinase, tachypnea, and altered mental status without any other clear etiology. Treatment involves stopping the antipsychotic medication and providing supportive care (to maintain hydration, treat fevers, and support cardiovascular, renal, and other organ functions).

Non-pharmacological Treatments

A large number of non-pharmacological treatments have been developed for schizophrenia and should be incorporated into a comprehensive treatment plan.[10] Individuals experiencing a first-episode of psychosis should be treated by a coordinated specialty care program (a clinic or treatment team specializing in first-episode interventions). Additional interventions should include cognitive behavioral therapy for psychosis, supportive psychotherapy, psychoeducation, cognitive remediation, social skills training, and supported employment services. For individuals who have poor engagement with services and thus experience frequent relapses or social disruption (eg, housing instability or legal problems), Assertive Community Treatment should be used (a multidisciplinary team that can engage patients in their homes or other community settings). Family interventions are indicated for individuals who have ongoing contact with family members. The amount and sequence of these interventions will depend on the individual's recovery goals.

SCHIZOPHRENIA AND SAFETY CONSIDERATIONS
Suicide Risk

Suicide risk is increased among patients with schizophrenia. Although statistics vary, it is estimated that approximately 5% to 13% of patients with schizophrenia die by suicide.[11] Risk factors include being male, identifying as Caucasian, having higher intelligence scores, living alone or not with family, experiencing recent loss events, having prior suicide attempts, and reporting a family history of depression.[12] Suicide is less associated with psychotic symptoms and more closely correlated with affective symptoms, psychomotor agitation, and awareness of one's illness.[11] Previous suicidal behavior is such a significant predictor among patients with schizophrenia who ultimately completed suicide that Pompili found 93% of that cohort had engaged in prior suicidal behavior.[11] Command auditory hallucinations are of particular concern to clinicians as the patients are assumed to be at a higher risk for obeying the hallucinatory commands. However, the presence of such command auditory hallucinations was not demonstrated to confer a significantly higher risk for suicide versus patients with schizophrenia without such commanding perceptual disturbances.[13] Age is also a risk factor, with the suicide risk for young adults with schizophrenia being three times higher than the risk for adults with schizophrenia.[11]

Evidence supports screening patients for suicide risk routinely. In one study, an estimated 49% of psychiatric patients (with mixed diagnoses) who completed suicide received care within the 4 weeks leading up to the suicide.[14] Standardized tools such as the Columbia-Suicide Severity Rating Scale can facilitate screening and assessment of suicide risk.[15]

As mentioned previously, clozapine should be considered for patients at high risk of suicide. This medication has a United States Food and Drug Administration-approved indication for reducing the risk of suicide, largely after the InterSePT study found clozapine was associated with a 24% decrease in the hazard ratio for time to a suicide attempt or hospitalization to prevent suicide.[16]

Risk for Violence

Violence risk associated with schizophrenia has been a topic of much research and public attention, yet interpretations are complicated by the wide variety of symptoms and co-occurring disorders that may accompany schizophrenia. A 2012 study from the National Epidemiologic Survey on Alcohol and Related Conditions reported that 2.9% of patients with serious mental illness (schizophrenia included) committed violent acts between years 2 and 4 following the baseline assessment, compared with 0.8% of people with no serious mental illness or substance use disorder. In the same sample, 10% of people committed violent acts if both serious mental illness and substance use were co-occurring.[17] Another landmark study, the MacArthur Violence Risk Assessment Study demonstrated that only two clinical symptoms were associated with violent acts in psychiatric patients after discharge: command auditory hallucinations and psychopathy. Although these two highly cited studies offer some evidence describing violence risk, predicting violence risk for an individual patient with schizophrenia remains a difficult task. Although there is some evidence for the validity and reliability of violence risk assessment instruments in the psychiatric population, little evidence exists for the use of such instruments in patients with schizophrenia.[18]

Studies have suggested that medication adherence can reduce the risk of violence. Maintaining a positive therapeutic alliance with the patients—in addition to being valuable in and of itself—can perhaps lessen the likelihood of medication nonadherence, or at least facilitate early identification and close monitoring when patients discontinue medication.[19]

Risk for Being the Victim of a Crime

A growing body of evidence has also noted that persons with schizophrenia are at risk of being the victims of both violent and nonviolent crimes.[20–22] According to a 2005 study, 25.32% of patients with a diagnosis of severe mental illness had been victims of a crime in the 1-year period that was studied: a rate that is 11.8 times higher than the general population. Patients with severe mental illness were 140 times more likely to be a victim of personal theft compared with the general population.[23] Further study is needed to understand the pathways to victimization and what interventions can reduce vulnerability among this population.[24]

Inability to Care for Self

Persons with schizophrenia are sometimes hospitalized due to inability to care for self, a notion with a complicated history that is subject to various interpretations. In the 1975 Supreme Court case of *O'Connor v Donaldson*, the Court established the constitutionality of civil commitment for three reasons (danger to self, danger to others, and inability to care for self) and described the term "inability to care for self" as a state of being "hopeless to avoid the hazards of liberty" (O'Connor v Donaldson, 422 US 563 (1975)). Since this federal clarification, state policymakers and clinicians have continued to wrestle with the definition and application of inability to care for self. For example, North Carolina defines the phrase as "reasonable probability of his suffering serious physical debilitation within the near future unless adequate treatment is given…" and explains, "A showing of behavior that is grossly inappropriate to the situation, or of other evidence of severely impaired insight and judgment shall create a prima facie inference that the individual is unable to care for himself…" (N.C. Gen. Stat. § 122C-3(11)). Alternatively, Connecticut describes the phrase as "inability or failure to provide for his or her own basic human needs such as essential food, clothing, shelter or safety" (Conn. Gen. Stat. Ann. § 17a.495(a)). Idaho state law uses the language "inability to provide for any of his own basic personal needs such as nourishment, or essential clothing, medical care, shelter or safety" (Idaho Code § 66–317(13)). As the definition and terms of civil commitment differ by region, every clinician should be well-versed in the legal definitions and boundaries of civil commitment in the states or territories where they practice.

SPECIAL TOPICS IN SCHIZOPHRENIA
Schizophrenia and Substance Use

Repeated large-scale studies have shown that nearly 50% of patients with schizophrenia have a co-occurring substance use disorder.[25] The most commonly used substances among patients with schizophrenia are cigarettes, alcohol, cannabis, and cocaine.[26] There is strong evidence for the effectiveness of integrated treatment that combines the treatment of a patient's psychotic illness with their substance use disorder, preferably performed in a single program or by a single practitioner.[27,28] Dual-diagnosis Motivational Interviewing may enhance treatment engagement among persons with schizophrenia and substance use disorders.[29]

Schizophrenia and Decision-Making Capacity

Emergency clinicians are likely to encounter individuals with schizophrenia who refuse recommended medical or psychiatric interventions, which raises questions about decision-making capacity among this patient population. It is important to keep in mind that schizophrenia affects each individual differently, so broad conclusions are problematic. Nevertheless, some key principles apply.

Medical decision-making ability (capacity) is related to one specific medical decision at one discrete time during which the evaluation is taking place. During a capacity assessment, the totality of the person's understanding of the issue and the person's cognitive abilities should be fully examined. For a person to demonstrate capacity (whether or not a mental illness is present), the person must meet four key measures: the ability to communicate a choice, the ability to understand the relevant information involved in the decision, the ability to appreciate the situation and its consequences, and the ability to reason about treatment options.[30] A review by Jeste and colleagues demonstrated that 10% to 52% of people with schizophrenia, compared with 0% to 18% of nonpsychiatric controls were classified as not having capacity.[31] The large percentage range, in addition to the overlapping rates, illustrates that a diagnosis of schizophrenia alone does not by itself indicate whether the patient has decision-making capacity.

SUMMARY

Although there remains much work to be done to elucidate further the causes of schizophrenia and other psychotic disorders and to develop preventive and disease-modifying interventions, it is also undeniably true that considerable progress has been made in recent decades that has advanced the scientific understanding of these disorders and created evidence-based treatments that are measurably beneficial for persons with these disorders.

Emergency physicians may be vulnerable to feeling frustrated or intimidated by schizophrenia and other chronic psychotic disorders if they only encounter affected patients during moments of acute crisis or primarily see the most chronic and refractory cases. Emergency physicians should keep in mind that there are countless others whose illness is well-managed, who are living full and productive lives in the community, and who will hardly ever visit the ED.

Although the patient with an acute exacerbation of schizophrenia or another psychotic disorder is likely to have different immediate needs than the patient with an acute coronary syndrome, a cerebral vascular accident, or a major trauma, it is no less of a health care emergency. ED teams that provide a safe place and rapid access to psychiatric evaluation and care provide a critically important service to patients, their families, and the community.

CLINICS CARE POINTS

- Schizophrenia is a clinical syndrome that often includes positive symptoms (eg, hallucinations, delusions), negative symptoms (eg, avolition), and disorganization (illogical thoughts or speech).

- Schizophrenia is differentiated from other psychotic disorders by its time course, associated features, and symptom severity.

- Treatment involves D2 antagonists (antipsychotic medication) accompanied by clinical monitoring for treatment effectiveness and adverse effects. Non-pharmacological therapies (psychotherapy, social skills training, family therapy) are of great value.

- When selecting an antipsychotic medication, clinicians should be guided by patient preference, treatment history, and recovery goals.

- Clinicians should remain alert for suicide risk factors, because persons with schizophrenia are at markedly increased risk of suicide compared with the general population.

- Having a diagnosis of schizophrenia may or may not affect medical decision-making capacity. A thorough capacity assessment should always be performed when patients refuse recommended treatment.

DISCLOSURES

The authors have no conflicts of interest to report.

REFERENCES

1. Moreno-Küstner B, Martin C, Pastor L. Prevalence of psychotic disorders and its association with methodological issues: a systematic review and meta-analysis. PLoS One 2018;13(4):e0195687.
2. Hooker EA, Mallow PJ, Oglesby MM. Characteristics and Trends of Emergency Department Visits in the United States (2010-2014). J Emerg Med 2019;56(3): 344–51.
3. Albert M, McCaig LF. Emergency department visits related to schizophrenia among adults aged 18-64: United States, 2009-2011. *NCHS data brief, no 215.* Hyattsville, MD: National Center for Health Statistics; 2015.
4. American Psychiatric Association. Diagnostic and Statistical Manual of Mental Disorders. In: Text Revision. Fifth Edition. American Psychiatric Association; 2022.
5. Lieberman JA, First MB. Psychotic Disorders. N Engl J Med 2018;379:270–80.
6. Sonnenschein SF, Gomes FV, Grace AA. Dysregulation of midbrain dopamine system and the pathophysiology of schizophrenia. Front Psychiatry 2020; 11(613).
7. Zamanpoor M. Schizophrenia in a genomic era: a review from the pathogenesis, genetic and environmental etiology to diagnosis and treatment insights. Psychiatr Genet 2020;30:1–9.
8. Opler M, Charap J, Greig A, et al. Environmental risk factors and schizophrenia. Int J Ment Health 2013;42(1):23–32.
9. Sideli L, Quigley H, La Cascia C, et al. Cannabis Use and the Risk for Psychosis and Affective Disorders. J Dual Diagn 2020;16(1):22–42.
10. American Psychiatric Association. American psychiatric association practice guideline for the treatment of patients with schizophrenia. 3rd edition. Washington, DC: American Psychiatric Association; 2021.
11. Pompili M, Amador XF, Girardi P, et al. Suicide risk in schizophrenia: learning from the past to change the future. Ann Gen Psychiatr 2007;6(10).
12. Hawton K, Sutton L, Haw C, et al. Schizophrenia and suicide: Systematic review of risk factors. Br J Psychiatry 2018;187(1):9–20.
13. Harkavy-Friedman JM, Kimhy D, Nelson EA, et al. Suicide attempts in schizophrenia: the role of command auditory hallucinations for suicide. J Clin Psychiatry 2003;64(8):871–4.
14. Burgess P, Pirkis J, Morton J, et al. Lessons from a comprehensive clinical audit of users of psychiatric services who committed suicide. Psychiatr Serv 2000; 51(12):1555–60.
15. Posner K, Brown GK, Stanley B, et al. The Columbia-Suicide Severity Rating Scale: initial validity and internal consistency findings from three multisite studies with adolescents and adults. Am J Psychiatr 2011;168(12):1266–77.
16. Alphs L, Anand R, Islam MZ, et al. The international suicide prevention trial (inter-SePT): rationale and design of a trial comparing the relative ability of clozapine and olanzapine to reduce suicidal behavior in schizophrenia and schizoaffective patients. Schizophr Bull 2004;30(3):577–86.
17. Van Dorn R, Volavka J, Johnson N. Mental disorder and violence: is there a relationship beyond substance use? Soc Psychiatr Psychiatr Epidemiol 2012;47(3): 487–503.

18. Singh JP, Serper M, Reinharth J, et al. Structured assessment of violence risk in schizophrenia and other psychiatric disorders: a systematic review of the validity, reliability, and item content of 10 available instruments. Schizophr Bull 2011; 37(5):899–912.
19. McCabe R, Bullenkamp J, Hansson L, et al. The Therapeutic Relationship and Adherence to Antipsychotic Medication in Schizophrenia. PLoS One 2012;7(4).
20. Maniglio R. Severe mental illness and criminal victimization: a systematic review. Acta Psychiatr Scand 2009;119(3):180–91.
21. Short TBR, Thomas S, Luebbers S, et al. A case-linkage study of crime victimisation in schizophrenia-spectrum disorders over a period of deinstitutionalisation. BMC Psychiatr 2013;13(66).
22. Wehring HJ, Carpenter WT. Violence and Schizophrenia. Schizophr Bull 2011; 37(5):877–8.
23. Teplin LA, McClelland GM, Abram KM, et al. Crime victimization in adults with severe mental illness: comparison with the National Crime Victimization Survey. Arch Gen Psychiatr 2005;62(8):911–21.
24. Fitzgerald PB, de Castella AR, Filia KM, et al. Victimization of patients with schizophrenia and related disorders. Aust N Z J Psychiatr 2005;39(3):169–74.
25. Green AI, Drake RE, Brunette MF, et al. Schizophrenia and Co-Occurring Substance Use Disorder. Am J Psychiatr 2007;164(3):402–8.
26. Khokhar JY, Dwiel LL, Henricks AM, et al. The link between schizophrenia and substance use disorder: A unifying hypothesis. Schizophr Res 2018;194:78–85.
27. McGovern MP, Chantal Lambert-Harris C, Gotham HJ, et al. Dual diagnosis capability in mental health and addiction treatment services: An assessment of programs across multiple state systems. Admin Policy Ment Health 2014;41(2): 205–14.
28. Drake RE, Essock SM, Shaner A, et al. Implementing dual diagnosis services for clients with severe mental illness. Psychiatr Serv 2001;52(4):469–76.
29. Martino S, Carroll K, Kostas D, et al. Dual Diagnosis Motivational Interviewing: a modification of Motivational Interviewing for substance-abusing patients with psychotic disorders. J Subst Abuse Treat 2002;23(4):297–308.
30. Appelbaum PS. Assessment of Patients' Competence to Consent to Treatment. N Engl J Med 2007;357(18):1834–40.
31. Jeste DV, Depp CA, Palmer BW. Magnitude of impairment in decisional capacity in people with schizophrenia compared to normal subjects: an overview. Schizophr Bull 2006;32(1):121–8.

Overview of Depression

Samantha Chao, MD, HEC-C

KEYWORDS

- Depression • Mood disorder • Psychiatric emergency • Suicide
- Depressive disorder

KEY POINTS

- Depressive disorders encompass a spectrum of diagnoses that differ in duration, timing, and etiology.
- Patients with depressive disorders are at higher risk for suicidality.
- Depressive disorders are more prevalent in women and transgender individuals.
- An underlying medical disorder, substance use, and other underlying psychiatric disorder must be excluded to make a primary diagnosis of major depressive disorder.
- Disposition planning depends primarily on assessing the patient's risk of harming themself, harming those around them, or an inability to care for themself.

INTRODUCTION

Depression and depressive symptoms are a common chief concern for patients presenting to the emergency department (ED). An analysis of emergency department visits in the United States between 2014 and 2016 estimated that 11.4% of all visits were related to depression.[1] The number of these visits is also steadily increasing.[2] Depression is a major risk factor for suicide,[3,4] one of the leading causes of death in the United States.[5] Our own trainees and colleagues can also be affected with growing attention to the prevalence of depression and suicide within the physician and health care worker community as a whole.[6,7]

DIAGNOSIS

What is colloquially referred to as "depression" is better described as a spectrum of depressive disorders distinguished by differences in duration, timing, and etiology.[4] Although there can be some overlap between depressive disorders and other mood disorders such as bipolar disorder, this article will focus on disorders with depressive symptoms as their primary feature (also called *unipolar depression*). Specifically, depressive disorders all share "the presence of sad, empty, or irritable mood."[4]

Department of Emergency Medicine, University of Michigan, TC-B1-380, 1500 East Medical Center Drive, Ann Arbor, MI 48109-5000, USA
E-mail address: skchao@umich.edu

Emerg Med Clin N Am 42 (2024) 105–113
https://doi.org/10.1016/j.emc.2023.06.013
0733-8627/24/© 2023 Elsevier Inc. All rights reserved.

Furthermore, to diagnose any of the depressive disorders, symptoms must impair a patient's ability to function.

The primary depressive disorders include disruptive mood dysregulation disorder (in pediatric patients), episodic depression, recurrent brief depression, persistent depressive disorder (also called *dysthymia*), and major depressive disorder. There are also etiology-specific depressive disorders, including premenstrual dysphoric disorder, substance/medication-induced depressive disorder, and depressive disorder due to another medical condition. The Diagnostic and Statistical Manual of Mental Disorders, Fifth Edition, Text Revision (DSM-5-TR) lays out the accepted American Psychiatric Association diagnostic criteria for major depressive disorder (**Table 1**). Note that important features include the presence of at least 5 specific symptoms nearly daily over a 2-week period that impair a patient's functioning, and these symptoms cannot be due to underlying substance use, another medical condition, or other psychiatric conditions including schizophrenia and bipolar disorder. "SIG E CAPS" is a common mnemonic used in medical training to help recall the symptoms of major depression (**Box 1**).[8]

Fine-tuning a diagnosis and distinguishing between the different types of depressive disorders may not change a patient's disposition in the emergency department and often falls to our colleagues in Psychiatry. However, it is still important to understand the major thematic differences in depressive disorders. For example, disruptive mood dysregulation disorder is a diagnosis only made in pediatric patients, between the

Table 1
Summary of diagnostic criteria for major depressive disorder taken from the diagnostic and statistical manual of mental disorders, fifth edition, text revision (DSM-5-TR)[4]

Diagnostic Criteria	
A. At least 5 symptoms present nearly every day for a 2 wk period; must include (1) or (2)	1. Depressed mood 2. Markedly diminished interest or pleasure in activities 3. Significant unintentional weight loss or weight gain 4. Insomnia or hypersomnia 5. Psychomotor agitation or slowing 6. Fatigue or loss of energy 7. Feelings of worthlessness or excessive/inappropriate guilt 8. Diminished ability to think or concentrate or indecisiveness 9. Recurrent thoughts of death or suicidal ideation
B. The symptoms cause clinically significant distress or impairment in social, occupational, or other important areas of functioning	
C. The episode is not attributable to a substance or other medical condition	
D. At least one episode is not better explained by a schizophrenia spectrum or other psychotic disorder	
E. There has never been a manic or hypomanic episode	

Box 1
SIG E CAPS mnemonic for recalling the symptoms of major depressive disorder.

Symptoms of Major Depressive Disorder

*S*leep disturbance

*I*nterest (diminished)

*G*uilt or feeling worthless

*E*nergy (loss)

*C*oncentration difficulties

*A*ppetite (increased or decreased)

*P*sychomotor activity (agitation or slowing)

*S*uicidal ideation

Adapted from Jha M.K., Qamar A., Vaduganathan M., et al., Screening and management of depression in patients with cardiovascular disease: JACC state-of-the-art review, J Am Coll Cardiol, 73 (14), 2019, 1827-1845.

ages of 6 and 18 years. Short-duration depressive episodes and recurrent brief depression refer to episodes of depressive symptoms lasting less than 14 days. A diagnosis of persistent depressive disorder is made in patients with at least 2 symptoms of major depression for at least 2 years. The differences between these diagnoses are illustrated in **Fig. 1.**

PATHOPHYSIOLOGY

Although the pathogenesis of depression is not fully understood, it is felt to have multiple contributors, including biologic, developmental, and psychosocial factors. Current twin, sibling, and genetic studies suggest an underlying genetic vulnerability to developing depression as well as a familial component to the disease.[9] The epigenetic component—the interplay between a patient's developmental and psychosocial environment with genetic predisposition—is also critical. Various environmental stressors can have an impact on the development of psychiatric and mood disorders, including traumatic events, childhood adversity, low social support, marital problems, financial problems, and loss.[10]

From a physiologic and anatomic standpoint, many mechanisms have been proposed as contributing to the development of depression. Depression has been associated with decreased amygdala volume. The hypothalamic–pituitary–adrenal (HPA)

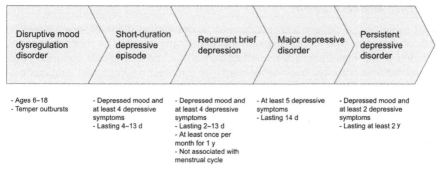

Fig. 1. Distinguishing between types of depressive disorders by diagnostic features, duration, and timing.[4]

axis, as the body's regulatory system for stress, may also play a role particularly in individuals with adverse childhood experiences and chronic stress. Multiple neurotransmitters have been implicated in depression, including deficiencies in monoamines (including serotonin and norepinephrine), glutamate, and γ-aminobutyric acid.[10] The majority of current first-line antidepressant therapies are directed at increasing serotonin and norepinephrine availability based on these prevailing theories; however, a more recent systematic review has called into question the strength of the evidence supporting serotonin's role.[11] Ultimately, there is still much to be learned about the complex mechanisms that contribute to the development of depression.

EPIDEMIOLOGY
Prevalence

Based on national survey data, 8.4% of adults in the United States had at least one major depressive episode in 2020.[12] Traditionally, studies have shown a higher prevalence in individuals identified as women, who experience an approximately 2-fold higher rate of major depression compared with individuals identified as men, particularly in adolescence.[4] Studies have also shown that there is a higher prevalence of major depression in transgender individuals compared with the general population in the United States and in other countries.[13–15] Major depression is more prevalent in adolescence; in 2020, it was most prevalent in individuals aged 18 to 25 years. This survey data further showed that those identifying with multiple (2 or more) races also had a higher prevalence of major depression.[12]

Risk Factors

As the pathogenesis of major depression is multifactorial, so too are the factors that put individuals at risk for developing major depression. Individuals with a first-degree family member with major depressive disorder are at a significantly increased risk for developing major depression. Negative affectivity is a well-established risk factor as these individuals are more likely to develop depressive symptoms in response to stressful life events. Adverse and traumatic childhood experiences also contribute. Furthermore, stressful events throughout a person's lifetime are known to precipitate depressive episodes. Certain social determinants of health are highly associated with major depression, including lower income, limited formal education, racism, and other forms of discrimination. The presence of another psychiatric disorder (ie, anxiety, substance use, personality disorders) is also a risk factor for developing depression.[4]

DIFFERENTIAL DIAGNOSIS
Underlying Medical Disorders

When evaluating a patient with concern for a depressive disorder, any underlying medical process that could explain the symptoms should be considered and excluded. These include an adverse effect from a medication (multiple commonly prescribed medications have been associated with depressive symptoms), metabolic issues such as hypothyroidism, and intracranial processes such as stroke or neoplasm. Chronic cognitive impairment, as seen in processes like dementia, can also mimic depressive-like symptoms.

Substance Use

Acute intoxication with various substances can lead to what appear to be depressive symptoms; however, if these symptoms resolve when the individual is no longer intoxicated, there is less concern for an underlying depressive disorder. Substance and medication-induced depressive disorders are a category in their own right. These are diagnosed in patients who develop prominent and persistent depressed mood in the setting of substance/medication use or withdrawal; these symptoms must also impair functioning.[4]

Other Psychiatric Disorders

Because management strategies can differ among the various mood and other psychiatric disorders, identifying the presence of disorders such as bipolar, schizophrenia spectrum, psychosis, and personality disorders is essential. Adjustment disorder is another potential explanation for depressive-like symptoms; it is a behavioral and emotional disturbance linked to an identifiable stress or stressors with symptoms lasting 3 to 6 months.

Appropriate Grief and Bereavement Response

Feelings of sadness, depressed mood, disturbed sleep, and disturbed appetite can be a part of a normal and healthy response to loss. Manifestations of grief may also differ culturally and generationally. An important differentiator between an appropriate grief response and major depression is that an appropriate grief response does not involve feelings of guilt, worthlessness, suicidal ideation, or significant functional impairment.[4,10]

INITIAL MANAGEMENT AND EVALUATION
History, Physical Examination, and Diagnostic Workup

Diagnosing a depressive disorder depends on a thorough history, including a psychiatric, family, social, and substance use history. Physical examination is important for a general assessment of the patient, including their mental status, and may also guide inclusion or exclusion of other differential diagnoses. Laboratory testing and imaging is used to evaluate for other underlying medical issues or alternative diagnoses such as substance intoxication.

Disposition

Disposition planning for a patient diagnosed with a depressive disorder involves deciding whether a patient can safely and reliably be followed in the outpatient setting or if they require the close monitoring and management of an inpatient admission. Our colleagues in Social Work, Case Management, and Psychiatry can often help provide resources and coordinate outpatient follow-up. Patients may follow up with their primary care doctor, a psychiatrist, a therapist, or any combination of these providers. There are also partial hospitalization and intensive outpatient programs, which intend to provide more rigorous and frequent outpatient psychiatric treatment.

Reasons to admit patients acutely presenting with a depressive disorder involve concern for imminent harm to themselves, imminent harm to others, or significant functional impairment such that the patient is not able to appropriately care for themselves. Thus, in addition to a thorough history and physical examination, evaluating a patient's risk for suicidality and homicidality is critical to determining the patient's ultimate disposition. ICAR2E and ED-SAFE[16] are validated screening tools emergency physicians can use to assess a patient's risk of suicide and self-harm; they take into account a patient's preexisting psychiatric diagnoses, a history of prior attempts, and access to lethal means. There are a variety of tools available to screen for potential violent and harmful behavior toward others; however, these tools have inconsistent predictive validity. Implicit biases on the part of the provider can also have an impact upon assessment of these risks in patients.[17]

Challenges with Disposition

Certain factors may make disposition planning for this population more nuanced and challenging. For example, it can be difficult to fully assess a patient presenting with suicidal ideation who is also acutely intoxicated. Patients may have an evolving or inconsistent report of symptoms and/or suicidal thinking during their visit particularly if the patient is aware that their symptoms influence whether admission or outpatient follow-up is recommended. Family members or other support persons may also be present; their level of concern about the patient's mental health may be greater than the patient's own, or they may provide collateral information that conflicts with the patient's reported history.

In all of these scenarios, re-evaluating the patient and taking collateral information into balanced consideration is prudent. When patients are intoxicated, their decision-making capacity is impaired, so expressions of suicidal intent may not reflect true autonomous preference. These patients should be reassessed when clinically sober, and at that time, risk assessments for safety planning can also be applied. For patients with symptoms that are inconsistent or conflict with collateral history obtained, establishing the likelihood of reliable follow-up and safety planning is key. Open communication, shared decision-making, and shifting the conversation toward understanding what the patient's and family's goals and concerns are can also obviate contentious dynamics. Using the assessment of consultants and other staff, including Social Work and Case Management, can also guide the primary emergency provider's decision-making.

It should further be noted that although pathways for outpatient and inpatient treatment seem clear-cut, there remain numerous barriers to obtaining outpatient mental health care, including affordability and availability of providers.[18] Boarding in the emergency department while awaiting transfer to an inpatient psychiatric facility is also a familiar and growing problem,[19] which has been exacerbated by the effects of the COVID pandemic on departmental flow.

Involuntary Admission

Some patients who require inpatient psychiatric treatment have decisional capacity and voluntarily consent to admission. Some patients do not wish to be admitted for treatment of a psychiatric disorder or refuse admission. In the United States, every state has laws that allow for involuntary admission of patients with an acute mental illness that may result in harm to self or others. These laws also allow for the patient to be held involuntarily within the emergency department until they can receive appropriate psychiatric treatment. The state laws vary in terms of hold duration, who can initiate the hold, and the rights of the patient being held.[17]

Antidepressant Therapy in the Emergency Department

Generally, it is safe to continue antidepressant or other mood-stabilizing medications that a patient is routinely prescribed while in the emergency department. Providers may also initiate therapies in consultation with psychiatric specialists. First-time initiation of antidepressant therapy in the emergency department, including selective serotonin reuptake inhibitors (SSRIs) and serotonin norepinephrine reuptake inhibitors (SNRIs), is controversial and requires careful consideration of the harms and benefits of initiating therapy. It can take up to 4 weeks for the majority of patients to experience a response to these medications.[20] Some data also suggest that initiating antidepressants may increase the risk of suicidality in children, adolescents, and adults less than age 25 years, leading to an FDA black box warning on these medications.[21] SSRIs and

SNRIs are also known to cause a variety of troubling adverse effects, including sexual dysfunction, nausea, changes in weight, and hypertension.

SPECIAL CONSIDERATIONS
Cultural Considerations

A syndrome similar to major depressive disorder can be identified across multiple cultural contexts, and within those contexts, the presenting symptoms of the disorder can vary.[4] Cultural humility and attention to the potential cultural factors affecting a patient's presentation can help prevent underdiagnosis of depressive disorders in these individuals.

Ethical Considerations of Suicide Intervention

In the Western conception of medicine and bioethics, respect for patient autonomy and a patient's preferences is often prioritized. The question becomes: How do we respond to a patient who voices a preference to die and what are our ethical obligations to that patient? This can be particularly pertinent in the emergency department setting where we evaluate patients not only with suicidal ideation but those in the aftermath of a suicide attempt.

A physician is ethically obligated to intervene when a patient attempts or threatens suicide.[22,23] The rationale is that suicidal patients may be experiencing acute psychiatric illness, which is impairing their decision-making capacity and influencing their conception of the harms and benefits of death. Treatment of the patient's psychiatric illness, including pharmacologic agents and therapy, may restore the patient's ability to make autonomous decisions and alter their initial desire for suicide.

A patient with decision-making capacity expressing an autonomous wish to die is its own complex and controversial ethical issue. It is a topic best explored by discussions surrounding the ethical justifications for and against physician-assisted death. The legality of physician-assisted death differs by state as well with current legislation allowing for it in 9 states (California, Colorado, Hawaii, Maine, New Jersey, New Mexico, Oregon, Vermont, and Washington) as well as the District of Columbia.[24,25]

Destigmatizing Mental Health

As evidenced by the various psychosocial and social determinant risk factors for developing major depression, those affected by depressive disorders and other psychiatric disorders are among the most socially vulnerable populations treated in the emergency department. Historical stigmatization of psychiatric disorders and mental health care have discouraged those suffering from mental health issues to seek help.[26,27] As one of the first-line responders to psychiatric emergencies, emergency department providers have the ability and responsibility to provide a safe and supportive environment for these vulnerable populations experiencing mental health crises. We can do so by being attentive to our language and attitudes when interacting with these patients as well as in our documentation and patient handoff.[28] Providers must also continue to be wary of implicit and explicit biases and how they may impact the care of our patients.

CLINICS CARE POINTS

- A diagnosis of major depressive disorder relies primarily on thorough history-taking.
- Laboratory testing and imaging can help exclude other underlying medical disorders leading to depressive symptoms.

- Initiating antidepressants, including SSRIs and SNRIs, in the ED setting is controversial and ultimately requires discussion of adverse effects and close outpatient follow-up.
- Health care providers have an ethical obligation to intervene when patients threaten or attempt suicide.
- Health care providers should be cognizant of environmental and psychosocial factors that make patients with depressive disorders a vulnerable population.
- Taking care with the language used when talking to and about these patients can prevent perpetuation of stigma and bias.

DISCLOSURE

The author has no conflicts of interest to disclose.

REFERENCES

1. Hill T, Jiang Y, Friese CR, et al. Analysis of emergency department visits for all reasons by adults with depression in the United States. BMC Emerg Med 2020;20(1):51.
2. Ballou S, Mitsuhashi S, Sankin LS, et al. Emergency department visits for depression in the United States from 2006 to 2014. Gen Hosp Psychiatry 2019;59:14–9.
3. Hawton K, Casañas I, Comabella C, et al. Risk factors for suicide in individuals with depression: a systematic review. J Affect Disord 2013;147(1–3):17–28.
4. American Psychiatric Association. Depressive disorders. In Diagnostic and Statistical Manual of Mental Disorders. 5th ed, Text Revision. American Psychiatric Association; 2022. Available at: https://doi-org.proxy.lib.umich.edu/10.1176/appi.books.9780890425787.x04_Depressive_Disorders. Accessed October 17, 2022.
5. Heron M. Deaths: leading causes for 2019. Natl Vital Stat Rep 2021;70(9):1–113.
6. Stehman CR, Testo Z, Gershaw RS, et al. Burnout, drop out, suicide: physician loss in emergency medicine, part I. West J Emerg Med 2019;20(3):485–94, published correction appears in West J Emerg Med. 2019 Aug 21;20(5):840-841.
7. Dutheil F, Aubert C, Pereira B, et al. Suicide among physicians and health-care workers: a systematic review and meta-analysis. PLoS One 2019;14(12): e0226361.
8. Jha MK, Qamar A, Vaduganathan M, et al. Screening and Management of Depression in Patients With Cardiovascular Disease: JACC State-of-the-Art Review. J Am Coll Cardiol 2019;73(14):1827–45.
9. Sullivan PF, Neale MC, Kendler KS. Genetic epidemiology of major depression: review and meta-analysis. Am J Psychiatry 2000;157(10):1552.
10. Zun L, Nordstrom K. Chapter 101: mood disorders. In: Walls R, editor. Rosen's emergency medicine concepts and clinical practice, vol. 2, 9th ed. Elsevier; 2018. p. 1346–52.
11. Moncrieff J, Cooper RE, Stockmann T, et al. The serotonin theory of depression: a systematic umbrella review of the evidence. Mol Psychiatry 2022. https://doi.org/10.1038/s41380-022-01661-0.
12. National Institute of Mental Health. Major depression. Updated January 2022. Available at: https://www.nimh.nih.gov/health/statistics/major-depression. Accessed September 6, 2022.
13. Reisner SL, Poteat T, Keatley J, et al. Global health burden and needs of transgender populations: a review. Lancet 2016;388(10042):412–36.

14. Nuttbrock L, Bockting W, Rosenblum A, et al. Gender abuse and major depression among transgender women: a prospective study of vulnerability and resilience. Am J Public Health 2014;104(11):2191–8.
15. Rotondi NK, Bauer GR, Travers R, et al. Depression in male-to-female transgender Ontarians: results from the trans PULSE project. Can J Commun Ment Health 2011;30(2):113–33.
16. ACEP Public Health and Injury Prevention Committee. Risk assessment and tools for identifying patients at high risk for violence and self-harm in the ED. ACEP. 2015. Available at: https://www.acep.org/globalassets/sites/acep/media/public-health/risk-assessment-violence_selfharm.pdf. Accessed October 17, 2022.
17. Baker EF, Brenner J, Chao S, Derse A, Marco C, Vearrier L. How to approach psych patients who refuse treatment in the emergency department. ACEP Now. May 12, 2022. https://www.acepnow.com/article/how-can-they-refuse/?singlepage=1. Accessed September 6, 2022.
18. Abar B, Holub A, Lee J, et al. Depression and anxiety among emergency department patients: utilization and barriers to care. Acad Emerg Med 2017;24(10):1286–9.
19. Nordstrom K, Berlin JS, Nash SS, et al. Boarding of mentally ill patients in emergency departments: american psychiatric association resource document. West J Emerg Med 2019;20(5):690–5.
20. Nierenberg AA, Farabaugh AH, Alpert JE, et al. Timing of onset of antidepressant response with fluoxetine treatment. Am J Psychiatry 2000;157(9):1423–8.
21. Friedman RA, Leon AC. Expanding the black box - depression, antidepressants, and the risk of suicide. N Engl J Med 2007;356(23):2343–6.
22. Beauchamp TL, Childress JF. Chapter 6: beneficence. In: Principles of biomedical ethics. 8th edition. New York, USA: Oxford University Press; 2019. p. 239–42.
23. Lo B. Chapter 40: ethical issues in psychiatry. In: Kiely J, editor. *Resolving ethical dilemmas a guide for clinicians*. 6th edition. Philadelphia, PA, USA: Wolters Kluwer; 2020. p. 292–8.
24. Lo B. Chapter 19: physician-assisted suicide and active euthanasia. In: Resolving ethical dilemmas a guide for clinicians. 6th edition. Wolters Kluwer; 2020. p. 146–56.
25. Britannica ProCon.org. States with legal physician-assisted suicide. Updated July 7, 2022. https://euthanasia.procon.org/states-with-legal-physician-assisted-suicide/. Accessed September 6, 2022.
26. Clement S, Schauman O, Graham T, et al. What is the impact of mental health-related stigma on help-seeking? A systematic review of quantitative and qualitative studies. Psychol Med 2015;45(1):11–27.
27. Hankir AK, Northall A, Zaman R. Stigma and mental health challenges in medical students. BMJ Case Rep 2014;2014. https://doi.org/10.1136/bcr-2014-205226. bcr2014205226.
28. Goddu A P, O'Conor KJ, Lanzkron S, et al. Do words matter? Stigmatizing language and the transmission of bias in the medical record. J Gen Intern Med 2018;33(5):685–91, published correction appears in J Gen Intern Med. 2019 Jan;34(1):164.

Bipolar Disorders in the Emergency Department

Carmen Wolfe, MD[a],*, Nicole McCoin, MD[b]

KEYWORDS

- Mania • Depression • Lithium • Affective disorder • Psychosis

KEY POINTS

- Patients with bipolar disorder have increased morbidity and mortality not only from psychiatric illness complications but also from organic medical illness, such as cardiovascular disease.
- Acute exacerbation of chronic bipolar symptoms may include a combination of symptoms of mania, depression, and psychosis.
- Always assess for suicidality in patients with any history of bipolar disorder.

EPIDEMIOLOGY AND PATHOPHYSIOLOGY

Bipolar disorders are defined by the *Diagnostic and Statistical Manual of Mental Disorders* (Fifth Edition; *DSM-5*) diagnostic criteria and include bipolar I disorder, bipolar II disorder, cyclothymic disorder, and other specified and unspecified bipolar disorders. Bipolar I disorder is defined by the presence of at least one manic episode and does not require other hypomanic, depressive, or psychotic episodes. Bipolar II disorder requires the presence of one hypomanic episode and one major depressive episode and excludes any patients with manic episodes.[1]

Onset of bipolar symptoms is predominantly early in life, with 69% of individuals experiencing their first symptoms before the age of 25.[2] Global lifetime prevalence for bipolar I disorder is 0.6% to 1.0%, and for bipolar II disorder is 0.4% to 1.1%.[3] Some data suggest that in the United States, up to 4.4% of the population will be affected at some point in their lives.[4] When comparing these two disease entities, individuals with bipolar II report more prominent depressive symptoms, higher socioeconomic status, higher functional status, and fewer hospitalizations.[5]

Bipolar disorders have high heritability, with twin studies reporting rates of 60%.[6] Genetic risk alleles have been identified and are shared among other psychiatric

a Department of Emergency Medicine, Tristar Skyline Medical Center, 3443 Dickerson Pike, Suite 230, Nashville, TN 37207, USA; b Department of Emergency Medicine, Ochsner Medical Center, 1514 Jefferson Highway, New Orleans, LA 70121, USA
* Corresponding author.
E-mail address: carmen.wolfe@hcahealthcare.com

Emerg Med Clin N Am 42 (2024) 115–124
https://doi.org/10.1016/j.emc.2023.06.014
0733-8627/24/© 2023 Elsevier Inc. All rights reserved.

disorders, with bipolar I having a higher association with schizophrenia than bipolar II.[7] Pathophysiology of the disease is incompletely understood, although changes in cellular function and brain structure have been observed in a process called neuroprogression. Factors promoting neuroprogression may include epigenetic mechanisms, mitochondrial dysfunction, inflammation, and oxidative stress.[8] MRI studies reveal reduced cortical thickness in the frontal, temporal, and parietal regions in bilateral hemispheres of patients with bipolar disorders.[9]

MORBIDITY AND MORTALITY

Patients with bipolar disorders use emergency services for a variety of reasons with more than two million visits in 2018 being coded as relating to bipolar disorder. The most common diagnosis assigned to these visits by *International Classification of Diseases, Tenth Revision* code were bipolar disorder, suicidal ideation, anxiety disorder, injury, and poisoning. Nearly half of these patients required admission, and aggregate emergency department (ED) charges for these visits was 738 million dollars.[10]

Mortalities of patients with bipolar disorder are elevated when compared with the general population. Life expectancy is decreased by 13.6 years for bipolar men, and 12.1 years for bipolar women.[11] Although increased suicide rates contribute to this disparity, a large population-based study in Denmark reveals that in this population it is primarily due to death from physical illnesses.[12] This suggests a need to help these patients focus on primary care for typical causes of death, such as cardiovascular disease.[13]

ACUTE PSYCHIATRIC PRESENTATION IN THE EMERGENCY DEPARTMENT
Mania and Hypomania

Mania and hypomania are characterized by increased activity or energy associated with three or more of the following symptoms: grandiosity, decreased sleep, pressured speech, flight of ideas, distractibility, increased goal-directed activity, psychomotor agitation, or excessive involvement in pleasurable activities with a high potential for painful consequences. For a diagnosis of mania, these symptoms must be present for a distinct period of at least 7 days, or any duration if symptoms are so severe that they require hospitalization. In addition, the symptoms must be significant enough to cause impairment in social functioning and must not be due to use of any substance. In contrast, a diagnosis of hypomania only requires 4 days of symptoms, and symptoms must not be significant enough to cause impairment in social functioning or to require hospitalization.[1] Patients who present to the ED with these symptoms should be identified and evaluated by psychiatry given the morbidity associated with acute manic episodes.

Depression

Major depressive symptoms are defined by the *DSM-5* to include depressed mood, loss of interest in almost all activities, significant weight loss or gain, sleep disturbance, psychomotor changes, fatigue, a sense of worthlessness, impaired ability to concentrate or make decisions, and recurrent thoughts of death.[1] Patients presenting with these symptoms may have previously been diagnosed with unipolar depression, but certain factors increase the probability that the patient has a bipolar disorder. These include earlier age of onset, psychosis, atypical depression with hyperphagia or hypersomnia, a family history of bipolar disorders, three or more previous depressive episodes, or abnormal responses to traditional antidepressant treatment, including the induction of hypomanic symptoms.[14] Patients presenting to the ED should be screened for these symptoms, and if symptoms have been present for more than 2 weeks, a major depressive episode should be suspected.

Psychosis

Psychosis is a defined by the presence of delusions or hallucinations without insight into their pathologic nature.[1,15] The presence of psychosis is common in patients with bipolar disorders and is associated with increased severity of symptoms and higher long-term morbidity.[16,17] Predictors of poor outcomes for these patients include poor premorbid functioning, Schneiderian delusions, younger age, and presence of psychotic symptoms during a depressive episode.[18]

Suicidality

Patients with bipolar disorder are at high risk for suicide, with rates up to 20 to 30 times greater than the general population. Among all major mood disorders, bipolar disease carries the highest risk of suicide.[19] Completed suicide is more common in bipolar II verses bipolar I.[20] Factors that increase risk for completed suicide include early onset of disease, a positive family history of suicide among first-degree relatives, previous suicide attempts, and other sociodemographic factors, such as age and male gender.[21] All patients with bipolar disorder should be screened for suicidal ideation with a detailed suicide assessment risk and safe disposition planning.

MEDICAL CLEARANCE OF PATIENTS WITH BIPOLAR DISORDER

Patients with bipolar disorder who present with severe psychiatric symptoms requiring hospitalization will require a thorough evaluation for medical conditions, which could cause or complicate their psychiatric symptoms.[22] This practice of medical clearance is familiar to emergency physicians, and special care should be taken among patients with bipolar disorder given their known comorbidities and medication toxicity profiles.

Hematologic Abnormalities

A complete blood count is important to rule out hematologic abnormalities. Carbamazepine is known to cause agranulocytosis, and divalproex is associated with thrombocytopenia.

Metabolic Disturbances

A basic metabolic panel should be performed to evaluate for electrolyte abnormalities. Lithium inhibits cyclic AMP formation in the renal tubules, therefore impairing the ability of the kidneys to concentrate urine. Excessive thirst or excessive urination may be noted by patients and should raise suspicion for nephrogenic diabetes insipidus, which may cause hypernatremia.[23] In addition, lithium may also cause elevated calcium levels secondary to hyperparathyroidism.[24]

Neurologic Abnormalities

Lithium has a narrow therapeutic window, and lithium toxicity must be suspected in any patient presenting with neurologic complaints. Mild toxicity is characterized by impaired concentration, lethargy, and slurred speech. Moderate toxicity progresses to confusion and unsteady gait. Severe toxicity, associated with lithium levels greater than 2.5 mmol/L, is characterized by delirium, coma, extrapyramidal symptoms, and seizure. These patients may require hemodialysis.[23]

Akathisia is a common side effect of multiple antipsychotic agents, such as aripiprazole, asenapine, cariprazine, ziprasidone, and lurasidone.[25] Extrapyramidal side effects may be seen with chlorpromazine and risperidone.[25] Tremor may be present at therapeutic lithium levels and may be a side effect of divalproex.[23,25]

Dermatologic Abnormalities

Lamotrigine is a common maintenance medication for bipolar disorder and is associated with Stevens-Johnson syndrome (SJS). A careful skin examination along with examination of the mucous membranes should be pursued in any patient on this agent who presents with rash.[26] Carbamazepine is also associated with dermatologic abnormalities, most commonly a benign maculopapular rash, although it can include a severe anticonvulsant hypersensitivity syndrome or SJS.[27]

Complications of Metabolic Syndrome

A multitude of medications used for treatment of bipolar disorder can increase a patient's risk for metabolic syndrome and associated complications. Treatment with antipsychotic medications is associated with weight gain, hypertriglyceridemia, hyperglycemia, increased risk of diabetes, and increased low-density lipoprotein cholesterol levels.[28] These metabolic changes increase a patient's risk for cardiovascular disease and associated mortality. Care should be taken to query the patient for symptoms that might suggest an acute complication of these chronic illnesses.[14]

TREATMENT IN THE EMERGENCY DEPARTMENT

Evidence regarding efficacy of medications in the long-term treatment of bipolar disorders is lacking, with systematic reviews revealing no high- or moderate-strength evidence for any particular agent.[29] Low-strength evidence supports the use of lithium, as it increases time to relapse of symptoms, and therefore, lithium is the mainstay of maintenance treatment for bipolar disorder.[29] Common medications used in the spectrum of treatment are discussed later and listed in **Table 1**. Typically, the primary focus on the treatment of bipolar disorders in the ED includes short-term stabilization of acute psychiatric symptoms and ensuring safe disposition. If long-term treatments are addressed in the ED, it is advised to do so in concert with formal guidance by psychiatry.

Acute Mania Treatment

Treatment of acute mania or hypomania includes mood stabilizers and antipsychotic agents. Common mood stabilizers used for acute mania include carbamazepine and divalproex. A meta-analysis of available evidence revealed that antipsychotic agents may be more effective than mood stabilizers and identified haloperidol, risperidone, and olanzapine as the best available options.[30] Another meta-analysis found no differences in head-to-head comparisons other than superiority of risperidone over aripiprazole and valproate.[31]

Acute Depression Treatment

Care must be taken as utilization of antidepressants in patients with bipolar disorder may be associated with mood destabilization. This risk is greater with bipolar I than bipolar II, with increased frequency and severity of mood elevations in this setting.[32] Medications that are approved by the Food and Drug Administration for acute depression in this population include only cariprazine, lurasidone, olanzapine-fluoxetine, and quetiapine. Given these limited options, other combinations, including antipsychotics and mood stabilizers, are often used off label.[25] Selection of an agent should be done in conjunction with psychiatry consultation given the complexities of medication choice.

Table 1
Common pharmacologic interventions in bipolar disorder

Pharmacologic Interventions: Medication Characteristics

Class	Generic Name	Trade Name	Indication	Route of Administration	Initial Dose (mg)	Special Considerations
Typical antipsychotics	Haloperidol	Haldol	Acute mania; acute stabilization of agitation	PO, IM, IV	2–5 mg PO, 2-10 mg IM/IV	Extrapyramidal side effects; QTc prolongation; lowers seizure threshold; risk of neuroleptic malignant syndrome
	Droperidol	Inapsine	Acute mania; acute stabilization of agitation	IM, IV	1.25-2.5 mg IM/IV	
	Chlorpromazine	Thorazine	Maintenance	PO	25–50 mg PO	Similar risks to other typical antipsychotics listed plus additional anticholinergic effects and agranulocytosis
Atypical antipsychotics	Olanzapine	Zyprexa	Acute mania; acute stabilization of agitation; maintenance	PO, IM (disintegrating tablet)	2.5–10 mg PO, 5-10 mg IM	Significant weight gain and metabolic disease; sedation
	Risperidone	Risperdal	Acute mania; acute stabilization of agitation if tolerating po; maintenance	PO (disintegrating tablet, oral solution); IM depot available for maintenance	1-3 mg PO, 25 mg IM q 2 weeks	Hyperprolactinemia
	Ziprasidone	Geodon	Acute mania; acute stabilization of agitation; maintenance	PO, IM	20–40 mg PO, 10-20 mg IM	QTc prolongation
	Quetiapine	Seroquel	Acute mania; acute depression; maintenance	PO	25-200 mg PO	Somnolence; hypertriglyceridemia
	Aripiprazole	Abilify	Acute mania; maintenance	PO (tablet, disintegrating tablet),	10–15 mg PO, 400 mg IM q month	

(continued on next page)

Table 1
(continued)

| | | | Pharmacologic Interventions: Medication Characteristics | | |
Class	Generic Name	Trade Name	Indication	Route of Administration	Initial Dose (mg)	Special Considerations
	Asenapine	Saphris	Acute mania; maintenance	IM depot available for maintenance; SL	5-10 mg SL	Transdermal formulation has been approved for schizophrenia
	Cariprazine	Vraylar	Acute mania; acute depression	PO	1.5-3 mg PO	Particularly longer half-life than many other antipsychotic options
	Lurasidone	Latuda	Acute depression	PO	20-40 mg PO	
Anticonvulsants	Carbamazepine	Tegretol	Acute mania; acute depression	PO	100-200 mg PO	Agranulocytosis; aplastic anemia; cardiac toxicity; hepatotoxicity; SIADH; skin eruption, including SJS/TEN; AGEP; DRESS
	Divalproex sodium	Depakote	Acute mania	PO	250-500 mg PO	Thrombocytopenia; hepatotoxicity; pancreatitis; hyperammonemia; encephalopathy; skin eruption, including SJS/TEN and DRESS
	Lamotrigine	Lamictal	Acute depression; maintenance	PO	25-50 mg PO	Aplastic anemia; aseptic meningitis; skin eruptions, including SJS/TEN and DRESS

| Other | Lithium | Lithobid | Acute mania, maintenance | PO | 300–450 mg PO | Narrow therapeutic window; myocardial toxicity; bradycardia; ataxia; slurred speech; confusion; hypercalcemia; hypothyroidism; nephrogenic diabetes insipidus |

DISPOSITION

Safe disposition planning is imperative in patients with bipolar disorder who present to the ED for acute psychiatric symptoms. First, suicidality should be assessed as above, and if any concerns are noted that the patient may be a threat to themselves or others, patients should be placed on a psychiatric hold for further evaluation by a comprehensive psychiatric team. Alcohol abuse and deterioration from previous levels of functioning can predict increased risk even without stated suicidal intent.[33] Even in the absence of suicidality, consideration should be given to hospitalization depending on the severity of symptoms. Patients with bipolar disorder are at increased risk of arrest as compared with the general population, especially when acute mania or substance use is involved.[34] This further pushes the imperative to stabilize acutely manic patients in a hospitalized setting to protect them from actions that would have devastating future consequences.

SUMMARY

Patients with bipolar disorder represent a complex subset of patients with mental illness who have high recurrence of psychiatric symptoms, poor functional outcomes, and high suicide risk. Patients may present in the ED with symptoms that are secondary to organic causes of medical illness, exacerbation of chronic psychiatric symptoms, or side effects from treatment of bipolar disorder. Little evidence guides medication choice for treatment of acute psychiatric symptoms. Care must be taken to ensure safe disposition in this patient population and often requires coordinated care among emergency physicians, psychiatrists, and social workers.

CLINICS CARE POINTS

- Patients with acute exacerbation of bipolar disorder may present to the emergency department with symptoms of acute mania, agitation, psychosis, or depressive symptoms. A thorough psychiatric examination should be performed in each patient to determine if the patient is a threat to themselves or others. Appropriate steps should be taken to keep each patient safe.

- The presence of bipolar disorder as a comorbid condition increases morbidity and mortality, not only from the psychiatric disease and associated risks such as suicide but also from other medical illnesses or the side effects of the medications used to treat the bipolar disorder.

- The emergency physician should have a strong working knowledge of the antipsychotics that may be used on demand in the treatment of acute agitation.

- The emergency physician must have an understanding of the common medications used to treat acute mania and acute depression, as well as those medications used as maintenance therapy for bipolar disorder. The physician must be well-versed in the adverse effects associated with each one. This will require continuing education, as new antipsychotics and other medications are released frequently, each with their own indication, formulation, and side-effect profile.

DISCLOSURE

This research was supported (in whole or in part) by HCA Healthcare and/or an HCA Healthcare–affiliated entity. The views expressed in this publication represent those of the authors and do not necessarily represent the official views of HCA Healthcare or any of its affiliated entities.

REFERENCES

1. Diagnostic and statistical manual of mental disorders. In: DSM-5. 5th ed. Washington, DC: American Psychiatric Association; 2013.
2. Nowrouzi B, McIntyre RS, MacQueen G, et al. Admixture analysis of age at onset in first episode bipolar disorder. J Affect Disord 2016;201:88–94.
3. Merikangas KR, Jin R, He JP, et al. Prevalence and correlates of bipolar spectrum disorder in the world mental health survey initiative. Arch Gen Psychiatr 2011;68: 241–51.
4. Harvard Medical School, 2007. National Comorbidity Survey (NSC). (2017, August 21). Retrieved fromhttps://www.hcp.med.harvard.edu/ncs/index.php. Data Table 1: Lifetime prevalence DSM-IV/WMH-CIDI disorders by sex and cohort.
5. Tondo L, Miola A, Pinna M, et al. Differences between bipolar disorder types 1 and 2 support the DSM two-syndrome concept. Int J Bipolar Disord 2022; 10(1):21.
6. Johansson V, Kuja-Halkola R, Cannon TD, et al. A population-based heritability estimate of bipolar disorder - In a Swedish twin sample. Psychiatr Res 2019; 278:180–7.
7. Cross-Disorder Group of the Psychiatric Genomics Consortium, Lee SH, Ripke S, et al. Genetic relationship between five psychiatric disorders estimated from genome-wide SNPs. Nat Genet 2013;45(9):984–94.
8. Berk M, Kapczinski F, Andreazza AC, et al. Pathways underlying neuroprogression in bipolar disorder: focus on inflammation, oxidative stress and neurotrophic factors. Neurosci Biobehav Rev 2011;35(3):804–17.
9. Hibar DP, Westlye LT, Doan NT, et al. Cortical abnormalities in bipolar disorder: an MRI analysis of 6503 individuals from the ENIGMA Bipolar Disorder Working Group. Mol Psychiatr 2018;23(4):932–42.
10. Eseaton PO, Oladunjoye AF, Anugwom G, et al. Emergency department utilization by patients with bipolar disorder: a national population-based study. J Affect Disord 2022;313:232–4.
11. Laursen TM. Life expectancy among persons with schizophrenia or bipolar affective disorder. Schizophr Res 2011;131(1–3):101–4.
12. Osby U, Brandt L, Correia N, et al. Excess mortality in bipolar and unipolar disorder in Sweden. Arch Gen Psychiatr 2001;58(9):844–50.
13. Kessing LV, Vradi E, McIntyre RS, et al. Causes of decreased life expectancy over the life span in bipolar disorder. J Affect Disord 2015;180:142–7.
14. McIntyre RS, Berk M, Brietzke E, et al. Bipolar disorders. Lancet 2020; 396(10265):1841–56.
15. World Health Organization. The ICD-10 classification of mental and behavioural disorders: clinical descriptions and diagnostic guidelines. Geneva: World Health Organization; 1992.
16. Keck PE Jr, McElroy SL, Havens JR, et al. Psychosis in bipolar disorder: phenomenology and impact on morbidity and course of illness. Compr Psychiatr 2003; 44(4):263–9.
17. Coryell W, Leon AC, Turvey C, et al. The significance of psychotic features in manic episodes: a report from the NIMH collaborative study. J Affect Disord 2001;67(1–3):79–88.
18. Carlson GA, Kotov R, Chang SW, et al. Early determinants of four-year clinical outcomes in bipolar disorder with psychosis. Bipolar Disord 2012;14(1):19–30.

19. Rihmer Z, Kiss K. Bipolar disorders and suicidal behaviour. Bipolar Disord 2002; 4(Suppl 1):21–5.
20. Rihmer Z, Barsi J, Arató M, et al. Suicide in subtypes of primary major depression. J Affect Disord 1990;18(3):221–5.
21. Plans L, Barrot C, Nieto E, et al. Association between completed suicide and bipolar disorder: A systematic review of the literature. J Affect Disord 2019;242: 111–22.
22. Tucci VT, Moukaddam N, Alam A, et al. Emergency Department Medical Clearance of Patients with Psychiatric or Behavioral Emergencies, Part 1. Psychiatr Clin 2017;40(3):411–23.
23. Price LH, Heninger GR. Lithium in the treatment of mood disorders. N Engl J Med 1994;331(9):591–8.
24. Naramala S, Dalal H, Adapa S, et al. Lithium-induced Hyperparathyroidism and Hypercalcemia. Cureus 2019;11(5):e4590.
25. Carvalho AF, Firth J, Vieta E. Bipolar Disorder. N Engl J Med 2020;383(1):58–66.
26. Schlienger RG, Shapiro LE, Shear NH. Lamotrigine-induced severe cutaneous adverse reactions. Epilepsia 1998;39(Suppl 7):S22–6.
27. Mehta M, Shah J, Khakhkhar T, et al. Anticonvulsant hypersensitivity syndrome associated with carbamazepine administration: Case series. J Pharmacol Pharmacother 2014;5(1):59–62.
28. Lieberman JA 3rd. Metabolic changes associated with antipsychotic use. Prim Care Companion J Clin Psychiatry 2004;6(Suppl 2):8–13.
29. Butler M, Urosevic S, Desai P, et al. Treatment for bipolar disorder in adults: a systematic review. Rockville (MD): Agency for Healthcare Research and Quality (US); 2018.
30. Cipriani A, Barbui C, Salanti G, et al. Comparative efficacy and acceptability of antimanic drugs in acute mania: a multiple-treatments meta-analysis. Lancet 2011;378(9799):1306–15.
31. Yildiz A, Nikodem M, Vieta E, et al. A network meta-analysis on comparative efficacy and all-cause discontinuation of antimanic treatments in acute bipolar mania. Psychol Med 2015;45(2):299–317.
32. Pacchiarotti I, Bond DJ, Baldessarini RJ, et al. The International Society for Bipolar Disorders (ISBD) task force report on antidepressant use in bipolar disorders. Am J Psychiatr 2013;170(11):1249–62.
33. Dutta R, Boydell J, Kennedy N, et al. Suicide and other causes of mortality in bipolar disorder: a longitudinal study. Psychol Med 2007;37(6):839–47.
34. Quanbeck CD, McDermott BE, Frye MA. Clinical and legal characteristics of inmates with bipolar disorder. Curr Psychiatr Rep 2005;7:478–84.

Recognizing and Responding to Patients with Personality Disorders

Jillian L. McGrath, MD[a,*], Maegan S. Reynolds, MD[b,c]

KEYWORDS

- Personality disorder • Personality trait • Cluster A • Cluster B • Cluster C
- Borderline • Countertransference

KEY POINTS

- Personality disorders are thought to occur in 15% of the general population and even more commonly in emergency department patients.
- The Diagnostic and Statistical Manual of Mental Disorders Fifth Edition recognizes 10 personality disorders, which are organized into 3 clusters (A, B, and C) based on shared diagnostic features.
- Personality disorders or traits create difficulty in clinical and interpersonal interactions, promoting missed diagnosis or underdiagnosis, nonadherence to medical recommendations, or other dangerous outcomes.
- Optimal management of individuals with personality disorders or traits requires the ability to be flexible and identify one's own emotions as they arise.

INTRODUCTION

Medical care for patients with personality disorders presents unique challenges with providers. The complexity of care is further amplified during an acute emergency department (ED) encounter. Personality disorders can prevent a clear diagnostic picture resulting in missed diagnosis or underdiagnosis of acute medical conditions. Such disorders can also create difficulty in clinical and interpersonal interactions, promoting nonadherence to medical recommendations or other dangerous outcomes.

Personality disorders are commonly seen in the ED. They are thought to occur in 15% of the general population, 40% to 60% of psychiatric patients, and are more

[a] Department of Emergency Medicine, The Ohio State University Wexner Medical Center, 750 Prior Hall, 376 West 10th Avenue, Columbus, OH 43210, USA; [b] Department of Emergency Medicine and Pediatrics, The Ohio State University Wexner Medical Center, Nationwide Children's Hospital Division of Emergency Medicine, Columbus, OH, USA; [c] Department of Emergency Medicine, 750 Prior Hall, 376 West 10th Avenue, Columbus, OH 43210, USA
* Corresponding author. Department of Emergency Medicine, The Ohio State University Wexner Medical Center, 750 Prior Hall, 376 West 10th Avenue, Columbus, OH 43210.
E-mail address: jillian.mcgrath@osumc.edu

Emerg Med Clin N Am 42 (2024) 125–134
https://doi.org/10.1016/j.emc.2023.06.015
0733-8627/24/© 2023 Elsevier Inc. All rights reserved.

frequent in ED users as well.[1] A study examining high frequency of ED use showed an overall increased rate of personality disorders in those patients (29.3%). This was even higher in those identified as 3-year consecutive high-frequency ED users (41.8%).[2] Patients with personality disorders also rely more heavily on psychiatric emergency services for continuity of care than patients with mood, substance use, anxiety, or psychotic disorders.[3] It is imperative for ED physicians and other providers to recognize and respond appropriately when a patient may have a personality disorder or traits impacting their presentation and management.

DEFINITIONS/BACKGROUND

Personality is defined as an enduring pattern of perceiving, relating, and thinking about the environment and oneself that is seen in a wide range of social and personal situations. The Diagnostic and Statistical Manual of Mental Disorders (DSM-5) specifically defines a personality disorder as an enduring pattern of inner experience and behavior that deviates markedly from the expectations of the individual's culture, is pervasive and inflexible, has an onset in adolescence or early adulthood, is stable over time, and leads to distress or impairment.[4] While an individual's personality is influenced by experiences, environment, and inherited characteristics, an individual's personality is considered relatively stable and predictable in ordinary situations. In the absence of disorder, personality is flexible, adaptable, and associated with mature coping strategies. When disordered, it is rigid, maladaptive, unpredictable, associated with immature or primitive coping strategies, and leads to stress and dysfunction for the patient and others. It is imperative to recognize a patient with a personality disorder or disordered traits. These disorders affect an individual's ability to function effectively in interpersonal settings. They also interfere with a variety of social circumstances, reduce treatment response for comorbid Axis I conditions, increase suicide rates, and may lead to substance abuse.[5]

DISCUSSION

Personality disorders are challenging to identify and diagnose. The DSM-5 recognizes 10 personality disorders, which are organized into three clusters based on shared diagnostic features. Although personality disorders are categorized by symptomatic clusters, they are also conceptualized as sharing a spectrum of genetic and environmental risk factors and underlying mechanisms. Cluster A personality disorders are characterized by common features of being odd and eccentric (paranoid, schizoid, and schizotypal personality disorders). Cluster B personality disorders are characterized by common features of being dramatic, emotional, and erratic (antisocial, borderline, histrionic, and narcissistic personality disorders). Cluster C personality disorders are characterized by common features of being anxious and fearful (avoidant, dependent, and obsessive-compulsive personality disorders).[4,5] Personality disorders may coexist; a patient may meet criteria for more than one disorder in addition to other psychiatric diagnoses.

The DSM-5 presents an alternative diagnostic model, the continuous dimensional model, that is expected to eventually replace the current categorical model (**Table 1**). The dimensional model views various personality features along several continuums. In this dimensional approach, personality disorders are assessed and diagnosed by measuring the level of functioning and pathologic traits within the personality. This model only contains 6 specific personality disorder types: borderline, obsessive-compulsive, avoidant, antisocial, schizotypal, and narcissistic. The two primary criteria assess the level of functioning and personality traits (along with standard

Table 1
Comparison of categorical vs dimensional model for diagnosis of personality disorders[10]

Categorical	Dimensional	
Cluster A	*Disorder types*	
• Paranoid	Antisocial	Narcissistic
• Schizoid	Avoidant	Obsessive-compulsive
• Schizotypal	Borderline	Schizotypal
Cluster B	*Trait domain*	*Personality functioning*
• Antisocial	Negative affectivity	Identity
• Borderline	Detachment	Self-direction
• Histrionic	Antagonism	Empathy
• Narcissistic	Disinhibition	Intimacy
Cluster C	Psychoticism	*Graded 0–4 on impairment*
• Avoidant	*Graded 0–3 on descriptiveness*	0 = little to no impairment
• Dependent	0 = not at all descriptive	1 = some impairment
• Obsessive-compulsive	1 = mildly descriptive	2 = moderate impairment
Personality disorder,	2 = moderately descriptive	3 = severe impairment
Unspecified	3 = very descriptive	4 = extreme impairment

requirement for stability across time, person, and place). Level of functioning is characterized by a degree of impairment in four areas within two domains. The domain of self is measured by identity and self-direction. The interpersonal domain is measured by empathy and intimacy. Functioning is graded on level of impairment ranging from mild to extreme. For a personality disorder to be diagnosed, patients must exhibit moderate to extreme impairment. The second component characterizes personality traits present. Patients are evaluated based on which traits in the following areas describe their personality, with each category having 3 to 6 sub-characteristic traits. The main trait domains are negative affectivity (vs emotional stability), detachment (vs extraversion), antagonism (vs agreeableness), disinhibition (vs conscientiousness), and psychoticism (vs lucidity). Each main trait domain is graded based on descriptiveness from none to very descriptive. Through grading under the level of function and personality traits, multiple main personality disorder types are able to be described on a continuum. Under this model, therapeutic interventions would focus most on the specific maladaptive areas.[1,4,6]

Categorical Model Clusters

Cluster A personality disorders: paranoid, schizoid, and schizotypal
Paranoid personality disorder. Paranoid personality disorder is marked by a pervasive distrust and suspiciousness of others (**Table 2**). Patients are reluctant to confide in other people or providers and have an underlying assumption that most people will harm or exploit them. In new situations, they search for confirmation of these expectations. They view even the smallest slight as significant and have a tendency to hold grudges. They tend to be socially isolated and avoid intimacy. They consider themselves to be rational and objective but outwardly may appear hypervigilant or unemotional with flat or restricted affect. When beliefs are challenged or a situation is stressful, patients may show profound anger, hostility, and referential thinking. The degree of paranoia is significantly higher than with schizoid and avoidant personality disorder. The prevalence of paranoid personality disorder in the general population is approximately 0.5% to 2.5%. There appears to be an increased incidence in families with schizophrenia and delusional disorder. The diagnosis is far more common in men than it is in women.[4,5]

Table 2
Characteristics of personality disorders from categorical approach[11]

Category	Disorder	Characteristics
Cluster A (odd/eccentric)	Paranoid	• Suspicious of others (assumes others will harm or deceive them) • Does not confide in others, socially isolated • Hypervigilant, unemotional
	Schizoid	• Detached from relationships and emotions • Prefers isolation • Does not care about opinions or emotions of others
	Schizotypal	• Odd beliefs outside cultural norms, distorted thinking • Peculiar and eccentric behavior • Uncomfortable in close relationships, social anxiety
Cluster B (dramatic/erratic)	Antisocial	• Disregard or violation of the rights of others • Repetitive unlawful acts, socially irresponsible behaviors • Does not show empathy or remorse
	Borderline	• Instability in relationships, splitting behavior • Rapidly shifting mood swings, impulsivity, intense emotions • Poor self-image, feelings of emptiness, repeated suicide attempts
	Histrionic	• Attention seeking, use physical appearance to draw attention • Excessive emotionality with emotional outbursts • Exaggerated mannerisms
	Narcissistic	• Egocentric, sense of entitlement, grandiose self-importance, ongoing need for admiration • Lack of empathy, due to ambition exploits others • Outwardly arrogant but inward self-esteem issues
Cluster C (anxious/fearful)	Avoidant	• Avoids social interactions or relationships, shy • Feelings of inadequacy, fear of rejection or humiliation, sensitive to criticism
	Dependent	• Submissive or clingy behavior • Fear of abandonment or being alone • Needs frequent reassurance from others, need to be taken care of
	Obsessive-compulsive	• Focus on details, order, perfection, and control • Inflexible, strict, and excessive standards • Willful behavior to maintain perfection and control

Schizoid personality disorder. Schizoid personality disorder is marked by emotional detachment and indifference to the world. Patients have little desire for relationships and limited emotional ties, even with family members. They express little or no discomfort over their detachment. With respect to employment, they prefer noncompetitive and isolative jobs with nonhuman themes (such as mathematics, philosophy, or astronomy). Solitary activities are not a source of discomfort. Thought processes are clear, and reality testing remains intact. Schizoid personality disorder affects about 7.5% of the population, with men diagnosed twice as often as women. As with paranoid personality disorder, the incidence of psychotic disorders in the relatives of these patients is higher, although this association is less robust.[4,5]

Schizotypal personality disorder. Elements of schizotypal personality disorder are cognitive, perceptual, and behavioral eccentricities and a pervasive discomfort with close relationships. Patients embrace unusual beliefs (such as telepathy, clairvoyance, and magical thinking) to a degree that exceeds cultural norms. They may appear socially uncomfortable or have excessive social anxiety. They may talk to themselves in public, and speech is often vague, digressive, or inappropriately abstract. The content of that speech may reflect ideas of reference, bodily illusions, and paranoia, but there is usually an absence of formal thought disorder, and their reality testing is intact. When acutely stressed, however, these patients may decompensate into brief psychotic states. Paranoid and schizoid personality disorders share many features of schizotypal personality disorder but differ by degree or absence of eccentricity. Schizotypal personality disorder affects about 3% of the population. There is no known gender ratio. There appears to be a higher occurrence of this disorder in the biological relatives of patients with schizophrenia and fragile X syndrome.[4,5]

Cluster B personality disorders (antisocial, borderline, histrionic, and narcissistic)
Antisocial personality disorder. Antisocial personality disorder is marked by repetitive unlawful acts, socially irresponsible behaviors, and a pervasive disregard for the rights of others. Antisocial behaviors develop early in adolescence. Patients may not conform to social norms and may be referred to as a "psychopath." Patients lack concern for the feelings and rights of others and do not show remorse or empathy. Patients may be charming and engaging, yet activities are characterized by illegal or deceitful pursuits, promiscuity, substance abuse, and/or aggressive or assaultive behavior. Antisocial personality disorder affects 3% of men and less than 1% of women. At least 75% of the prison population carries the diagnosis. Patients with this disorder have an onset of conduct disorder before the age of 15 and frequently suffer from comorbid conditions. This disorder occurs five times more commonly in first-degree relatives of men with the disorder. Antisocial personality disorder is the personality disorder most resistant to treatment although some improvement can occur during middle age.[4,5]

Borderline personality disorder. Borderline personality disorder (BPD) is marked by an impaired capacity to form stable interpersonal relationships. Other features include affective instability (rapidly shifting mood swings), impulsivity, identity disturbance (chronic boredom or emptiness), recurrent manipulative suicidal behaviors or self-mutilation, and idealization/devaluation (splitting). When faced with real or perceived separation, these patients often react with intense emotions of fear and anger. Under acute stress, borderline patients may also experience brief psychotic episodes or dissociative phenomena. BPD has extensive overlap with the histrionic, narcissistic, and dependent disorders, but individuals with these conditions tend to have more stable identities, and they rarely engage in self-mutilation or chronic suicidal behaviors. Bipolar spectrum disorders can be difficult to distinguish from those with BPD, as the two may coexist. Substance abuse disorders, especially alcohol abuse, have a major comorbidity with BPD. BPD is the most prevalent personality disorder in all clinical settings (12%–15%). It is believed to occur in 2% to 3% of the general population, with a 2:1 female-to-male ratio and is usually diagnosed before the age of 40 years. A high co-occurrence rate of major depressive disorder is observed in patients with borderline personality, but recent research suggests that rather than having coexisting disorders, the depression associated with borderline personality is reflective of the depressive nature of borderline pathology and the consequences of chaotic lifestyles. Some patients experience a marked decrease in their impulsive and self-injurious behaviors around middle age.[4,5]

Histrionic personality disorder. Histrionic personality disorder is characterized by excessive emotionality and need for attention. Patients are overly concerned with their physical appearance or attractiveness and may be inappropriately seductive with regard to dress or behavior. While they appear superficially charming, others tend to view them as vain or disingenuous. They have difficulty managing frustration and are prone to emotional outbursts. Speech may be vague or unfocused and mannerisms exaggerated. While histrionic and narcissistic personality disorders are often closely associated, other cluster B personality disorders remain in the differential diagnosis. Narcissistic PD patients are more preoccupied with grandiosity. BPD patients typically display more despair and suicidal behaviors, but there is a high comorbidity with histrionic and BPDs as well. Histrionic disorder occurs in 2% to 3% of the general population. Women receive the diagnosis more often than men. This disorder is more common in first-degree relatives of people with this PD. Some individuals experience an attenuation of symptoms in middle age.[4,5]

Narcissistic personality disorder. Narcissistic personality disorder is marked by an overwhelming self-absorption and egocentricity. Patients possess a grandiose sense of self-importance or uniqueness. They prefer to associate with people that they deem special or unique as well. Typically, individuals are ambitious to the point of being exploitative. They lack empathy for others and may break rules to meet their goal. They tend to react with extreme disappointment or rage when others' needs interfere with their desires. Although outwardly arrogant, the patient is prone to hypersensitivity and self-esteem issues. Therefore, even slight criticism may be met with intense emotion or rage. Other cluster B personality disorders often coexist. However, BPD patients are more impulsive, less organized, and have a less cohesive identity. Histrionic PD patients are more outwardly emotional. Antisocial PD patients focus on short-term material gain while narcissistic PD patients exploit people to maintain his or her grandiose self-image. Narcissistic PD occurs in less than 1% of the general population, although it is thought to be more prevalent among patients in various medical settings (2%–15%). Men are more frequently diagnosed with the condition. Comorbid mood disorders are common. The course of this condition is chronic, and patients are prone to severe midlife crises.[4,5]

Cluster C personality disorders: avoidant, dependent, and obsessive-compulsive
Avoidant personality disorder. Avoidant personality disorder is characterized by excessive discomfort with or fear of intimate relationships that results in avoidance of social interactions. In order to protect themselves against potential humiliation, rejection, or negative feedback, patients do not deviate from a safe and predictable daily routine. Patients appear awkward and shy and suffer from very low self-esteem and feelings of inadequacy. While genuinely desiring relationships, they are unwilling to enter into them because of real or perceived signs of humiliation, rejection,

or negative feedback. Patients with avoidant PD are able to function in relationships when the environment is considered safe and protective. Avoidant PD patients desire relationships with others, in contrast with schizoid PD. Avoidant personality disorder occurs in approximately 1% of the general population. There is high comorbidity with anxiety disorders and social phobia.[4,5]

Dependent personality disorder. Dependent personality disorder is marked by a clingy or submissive behavior. Patients have a strong desire for others to care for them and are preoccupied with fear of rejection or abandonment. Patients will placate others and go to extreme lengths to preserve relationships, even when physically or emotionally abusive. They may be overly agreeable or look to others for assurance about simple decisions. Compared with histrionic PD patients, BPD patients have shorter and more numerous relationships and express more affect and anger around real or perceived abandonment. Dependent personality disorder accounts for about 2.5% of all personality disorders, with women more commonly diagnosed than men. Patients with a history of childhood separation anxiety or chronic illness may be predisposed to the disorder. There is significant comorbidity with depressive disorders and substance abuse, and patients easily become victims of physical or emotional abuse.[4,5]

Obsessive-compulsive personality disorder. Features of obsessive-compulsive personality disorder are perfectionism, inflexibility, and need for control. Patients are preoccupied with rules, efficiency, details, schedules, and procedures. They may lose purpose or leave tasks uncompleted yet dislike delegating tasks or tend to micromanage tasks. They maintain an inflexible adherence to their own internally strict and excessive standards and are inflexible in their morals and values. Patients with obsessive-compulsive disorder have true obsessions and compulsions, whereas patients with the obsessive-compulsive PD have more willful behavior that tends to be praised or valued. This personality disorder is common in the general population, with men receiving the diagnosis more often than women. It is more common among first-degree relatives of patients with this disorder and has an increased concordance in identical twins. Obsessive-compulsive PD is one of the least impairing personality disorders, and patients with this condition often achieve success.[4,5]

Emergency department management. Management of personality traits and disorders is especially difficult in the ED setting. Patients may present in acute crisis situations. The stressful and chaotic environment of the ED may intensify the drivers of underlying personality traits and promote maladaptive communication or behavior. Personality disorders present in family members or others at a patient's bedside may also adversely affect patient care. Difficult patients in the ED, regardless of cause, can be overlooked or undertreated. It is recommended that physician and other care providers focus efforts on avoiding emotional escalations and minimizing the effect personality traits or disorders have on delivery of care.[1] Therefore, it is important to recognize patients with potential personality disorders and understand strategies to achieve optimal patient interactions and best possible medical outcomes (**Table 3**).

A thorough history is important, and necessary medical information should be gathered as efficiently as possible. The interview should be conducted in a calm and objective manner. Provide clear and factual information about diagnostic testing and treatment. In most cases, it is helpful to allow patients to participate in establishing a treatment plan. In patients with personality disorders, a variety of distractions are unavoidable and should be expected. For example, patients with cluster B traits may offer more extraneous details or make dramatic comments. Clinical encounters are

Table 3
Management strategies for treating patients with personality disorders in the emergency department setting[1,12]

Specific to Disorder Category	General Strategies
Cluster A: • Repeat interviews may be necessary with tendency to underreport • Show genuine curiosity and be factual • Use consistent, clear terminology that avoids the use of medical jargon • Respect patient beliefs while directly addressing beliefs that inhibit evaluation Cluster B: • May require repeated reassurance • Consistent communication from all team members; gather team for interactions • Be direct and avoid emotion • Set clear limits and boundaries early Cluster C: • May require repeated explanation of medical plan to optimize adherence • Show empathy, but be direct • Provide a stable and calming environment whenever possible	Remain objective; each visit is new and should focus on ruling out acute medical conditions Respect patients' privacy and needs Set clear limits early and manage expectations for evaluation and treatment Ensure clear and consistent communication among all team members Tailor the environment to the patient's needs whenever possible and provide appropriate reassurance Recognize biases and countertransference: • Understand the stigma associated with personality disorder diagnoses • Check for provider reactions to patients such as feeling criticized, mistreated, overwhelmed, overinvolved, overprotective, or helpless • Acknowledge biases or countertransference feelings and seek help from colleagues to provide optimal patient care

more likely to escalate in emotion. Patients or family may make accusations of the provider or various staff not being helpful or caring enough or try splitting behaviors. Patients with cluster C traits may require excessive reassurance or be indecisive with regard to history or treatment plans. Alternatively, patients with cluster A traits may underreport symptoms to avoid the interview or be mistrustful of the care team. An empathic approach to patients' fears or concerns is ideal. Offering validation to the difficulty of the ED experience is often helpful. Despite this, it is very common to witness escalation and misunderstandings in communication with providers. Stating your desire to help but that you as a provider may not be able to fix the problem at hand may help to maintain a productive therapeutic relationship. Providers may need to be proactive in setting expectations for the ED visit. At the onset of the encounter or at any point when a difficult situation escalates, providers should set clear limits in interventions and provide consistent messaging from all care team members regarding expectations.[1]

Although physicians and other providers should make note of personality disorder diagnoses, it is essential to acknowledge the "labeling" that may occur and negatively affect care for patients. Patients are very easily prejudged and biases applied. Evidence suggests that personality disorders might be even more stigmatizing than other psychiatric diagnoses. The belief that people with personality disorders should be able to control their behavior results in symptoms being viewed as manipulations or rejections of help. Patients may be viewed as difficult or poorly behaved rather than sick. The public reacts less sympathetically to individuals described as having a personality disorder and is less likely to think these individuals need professional help than those with other psychiatric disorders despite significant impairments these individuals experience.[1,7]

It is imperative to differentiate personality disorder symptoms from other acute medical and psychiatric conditions. There is significant comorbidity and diagnostic overlap with other psychiatric conditions. Coexistent personality disorders are especially common in mood disorders. A meta-analysis conducted to identify the proportions of comorbid personality disorders in mood disorders showed the risk of having at least one comorbid personality disorder was high across all three mood disorders. The highest risk of comorbid personality disorder was in dysthymic disorder (0.60) but still prevalent with bipolar disorder (0.42) and major depressive disorder (0.45). Cluster B and C personality disorders were most frequent in bipolar disorder, while cluster C personality disorders dominated in major depressive disorder and dysthymic disorder. Among the specific personality disorders, the paranoid (.11 vs. .07/.05), borderline (.16 vs. .14/.13), histrionic (.10 vs. .06/.06), and obsessive-compulsive (.18 vs. .09/.12) PDs occurred more frequently in bipolar disorder versus major depressive disorder/dysthymic disorder. The avoidant personality disorder (.22 vs. .12/.16) was most frequent in dysthymic disorder.[8]

Optimal management of individuals with personality traits or disorders requires the ability to be flexible and identify one's own emotions as they arise. Countertransference refers to the emotion or attitude induced in the provider toward patients. Countertransference describes the mental state that is induced in the provider, whereas cognitive bias refers to the preconceptions that individuals possess. Countertransference (feelings evoked or experienced by providers) can be objective (induced by patients' attitudes and behaviors) or subjective (stemming from provider experiences). The subjective feelings that health care providers tend to feel are typically long lasting, whereas objective feelings tend to be more transient and disappear quickly. The concern is that medical decisions are influenced by objective, transitional experiences. Research suggests that therapists' reactions may vary depending on the type of personality disorder they are treating. The patients' level of functioning was related to the type of countertransference experienced by the treating provider as well. Providers treating individuals with cluster A overall felt criticized or mistreated. Providers treating individuals with cluster B overall felt overwhelmed, inadequate, helpless, disorganized, and at times, overinvolved with their patients. For providers treating individuals with cluster C, the most common reaction is seeing patients as vulnerable or in need of protection.[1,9] Awareness of these potential biases or emotions and proactive identification and subsequent mitigation strategies are imperative for providers to give optimal medical care for patients with personality disorders.

SUMMARY

Personality disorders are challenging to recognize, diagnose, and manage even when care settings provide continuity. It is important to identify patients with potential personality disorders and understand strategies to achieve optimal patient interactions and best possible medical outcomes in the ED.

CLINICS CARE POINTS

- Disordered personalities are rigid, maladaptive, unpredictable, and associated with immature or primitive coping strategies, leading to stress and dysfunction for the patient and others.
- There is significant comorbidity and diagnostic overlap with other psychiatric conditions. Coexistent personality disorders are especially common in mood disorders.

> • Optimal management of individuals with personality traits or disorders requires the ability to be flexible and identify one's own emotions as they arise.

DISCLOSURE

The authors have no financial or other conflicts of interest to disclose related to this article.

REFERENCES

1. Moukaddam N, Araceli F, Anu M, et al. Difficult patients in the emergency department. Psychiatr Clin 2017;40(3):379–95. Copyright © 2017 Elsevier Inc.
2. Gentil L, Guy G, Helen-Maria V, et al. Predictors of recurrent high emergency department use among patients with mental disorders. Int J Environ Res Publ Health 2021;18(9):4559.
3. Richard-Lepouriel H, Weber K, Baertschi M, et al. Predictors of recurrent use of psychiatric emergency services. Psychiatr Serv 2015;66:521–6.
4. American Psychiatric Association, Diagnostic and statistical manual of mental disorders, 5th edition, 2013, American Psychiatric Association; Arlington, VA. Available at: https://doi.org/10.1176/appi.books.9780890425596. Accessed December 1, 2022.
5. Blais M, Smallwood P, Groves J, et al. Personality and personality disorders, Massachusetts General Hospital Comprehensive Clinical Psychiatry, 39, 2016, 433–444.e5.
6. Zimmermann J, Kerber A, Rek K, et al. A brief but comprehensive review of research on the alternative DSM-5 model for personality disorders. Curr Psychiatry Rep 2019;21(9):92.
7. Sheehan L, Nieweglowski K, Corrigan P. The stigma of personality disorders. Curr Psychiatry Rep 2016;18:11.
8. Oddgeir M, Monica K, Sabine Ø, et al. Comorbidity of personality disorders in mood disorders: a meta-analytic review of 122 studies from 1988 to 2010. Journal of Affective Disorders Friborg 2013;145(2). 2012.
9. Colli A, Tanzilli A, Dimaggio G, et al. Patient personality and therapist response: an empirical investigation. Am J Psychiatry 2014;171:102–8.
10. Andrew Skodol, "Dimensional-categorical approach to assessing personality disorder pathology," Uptodate.com, 2021. Available at: https://www.uptodate.com/contents/dimensional-categorical-approach-to-assessing-personality-disorder-pathology. Accessed February 7, 2023.
11. Available at: https://www.psychiatry.org/patients-families/personality-disorders/what-are-personality-disorders. Accessed February 7, 2023.
12. Moukaddam N, AufderHeide E, Flores A, et al. Shift, interrupted: strategies for managing difficult patients including those with personality disorders and somatic symptoms in the emergency department. Emerg Med Clin North Am 2015;33(4):797–810.

Geriatric Psychiatric Emergencies

Michelle A. Fischer, MD, MPH[a],*, Monica Corsetti, MD[b]

KEYWORDS

- Geriatrics • Elderly • Delirium • Psychiatric emergencies • Dementia • Depression

KEY POINTS

- The US Census Bureau reports a steady increase in the population aged 65 and older with a 36% increase over the ten-year period from 2009 to 2019. As of 2020, this age group encompasses approximately 17% of the US population.
- Delirium carries a high mortality rate for the geriatric population and is often under-recognized.
- Psychiatric symptoms in the geriatric population are often a manifestation of an organic illness.
- Additional history sources are often necessary when evaluating a geriatric patient with altered mental status in the Emergency Department (ED).
- Antipsychotics are first-line treatments for geriatric patients experiencing acute delirium when non-pharmacologic interventions are inadequate.

INTRODUCTION
Epidemiology

Geriatric patients are defined as those more than the age of 65 years of age according to the American Geriatrics Society.[1] The geriatric population is the fastest-growing age group in the United States; the 2010 US census noted that the population of patients 85 years of age and older is increasing at three times the rate of the overall US population.[1] The geriatric patient in the Emergency Department (ED) presents unique challenges in evaluation, diagnosis, and management. Older adults may have dementia (or other reasons for cognitive decline) at baseline, making the recognition of a true psychiatric emergency difficult. One 2022 study that looked at cognitive impairment in the US estimates the prevalence of dementia in those over the age of 65 to be 10% with minor cognitive impairment existing in 22%.[2] This means that 1 in 10 ED patients'

a Penn State Health Milton S. Hershey Medical Center, 500 University Drive, Hershey, PA 17033, USA; b Penn State Health Holy Spirit Medical Center, 503 N. 21st Street, Camp Hill, PA 17011, USA
* Corresponding author. Penn State Milton S. Hershey Medical Center, Department of Emergency Medicine, 500 University Drive, MC H043, Hershey, PA 17033.
E-mail address: mfischer1@pennstatehealth.psu.edu

Emerg Med Clin N Am 42 (2024) 135–149
https://doi.org/10.1016/j.emc.2023.06.016
0733-8627/24/Published by Elsevier Inc.
emed.theclinics.com

cases over the age of 65 may be confounded by baseline cognition deficits. It is also well-documented that the prevalence of dementia increases with age. The incidence of dementia is 35% in those more than the age of 90. These realities further blur the presentation between a true psychiatric disease process versus an organic one. Furthermore, delirium is extremely common in geriatric ED patients, occurring at a rate as high as 10%. Unfortunately, it is too often an under-recognized diagnosis with one study estimating that Emergency physicians miss delirium in as many as 57% to 83% of cases.[3] The consequences of missing true geriatric psychiatric emergencies, such as delirium, carry an extremely high mortality rate.

Delirium

When evaluating elderly patients with a psychiatric emergency, it is important to recognize potential cases of delirium and to differentiate between delirium and dementia. *Delirium*–as summarized from the fifth edition of the Diagnostic and Statistical Manual of the American Psychiatric Association (DSM-5) – is a disturbance in attention and awareness that develops over a brief period, represents an acute change from baseline attention and awareness, and tends to fluctuate in severity throughout the day. Delirium also involves a disturbance in cognition and is not better explained by a pre-existing neurocognitive disorder or a severely reduced level of arousal, such as coma.[4] Failure to recognize delirium contributes to not only increased morbidity and mortality but also increased cost and length of hospital stay.[5] It should be noted that 3 different subtypes of delirium exist: hypoactive, hyperactive, and mixed psychomotor. The hypoactive subtype of delirium patient displays decreased activity and withdrawn behavior. This subtype is the most common, has the highest mortality, and is the most often missed subtype of delirium. In contrast, the hyperactive subtype patient is agitated and aggressive. The mixed psychomotor subtype displays features of both.[6,7] **Table 1** summarizes several clinical misconceptions about delirium and the current evidence refuting the misconception.

Dementia

Dementia, by contrast, is often insidious in onset, does not tend to fluctuate in severity, and does not present with alterations in attention and consciousness.[1] It is important to emphasize that a patient with underlying dementia may present with acute delirium and that the two processes are not mutually exclusive. Additionally, dementia with neurocognitive impairment is common in elderly patients, affecting 10% of those over the age of 65 and 35% over the age of 90.

The aging process brings several life changes that may affect mental health, including failing physical health, loss of a loved one, or decreased mobility and social interaction. With these life experiences, patients may develop loneliness, grief, or social isolation. When these feelings become more constant than transitory, they can lead to mental illness such as anxiety or depression. Although 1 in 4 older adults experience mental health disorders such as depression, anxiety, or dementia, true mental emergencies in this population are most often the result of an organic process. *Altered mental status and psychiatric symptoms are common manifestations of organic processes.* A true psychiatric cause of a new psychosis is rare in the geriatric population,[6] and other diagnoses should be considered and eliminated prior to labeling the patient's illness as purely psychiatric in nature.

Depression and Suicide

Depression is the most prevalent and common psychiatric disorder in the geriatric population with estimates that range from 5 to 56%.[10] Depression is not a normal

Table 1
Ten delirium misconceptions juxtaposed with best evidence[8,9]

Misconception	Best Evidence
This patient is oriented to person, place, and time. They are not delirious.	Delirium evaluation minimally requires assessing attention, orientation, memory, and the thought process, ideally at least once per nursing shift, to capture daily fluctuations in mental status.
Delirium always resolves.	Especially in cognitively vulnerable patients, delirium may persist for days or even months after the proximal "causes" have been addressed.
Frail, older patients get confused at times, especially after receiving pain medication.	Confusion in frail, older patients always requires further assessment.
The goal of a delirium work-up is to find the main cause of delirium.	Delirium etiology is typically multifactorial.
New-onset psychotic symptoms in late life likely represent primary mental illness.	New delusions or hallucinations, particularly nonauditory, in middle age or later deserve evaluation for delirium or another medical cause.
Delirium in patients with dementia is less important because these patients are already confused at baseline.	Patients with dementia deserve even closer monitoring for delirium because of their elevated delirium risk and because delirium superimposed on dementia indicates marked vulnerability.
Delirium treatment should include psychotropic medication.	The role of psychotropic medications in delirium remains unclear. They are best used judiciously, if at all, for specific behaviors or symptoms rather than delirium itself.
The patient is delirious due to a psychiatric cause.	Delirium always has a physiological cause.
It is often best to let quiet patients rest.	Hypoactive delirium is common and often under-recognized.
Patients become delirious just from being in the Intensive care unit.	Delirium in the intensive care unit, as with delirium occurring in any setting, is caused by physiological and pharmacological insults.

part of aging, but it is a frequent and undertreated problem of aging and is even more prevalent in elderly patients with underlying dementia. The relationship between depression and dementia is still an active area of research to fully understand how they coexist. It is known that older patients with depression are more likely to develop dementia and that those with dementia are more likely to become depressed. The risk of suicide parallels this high prevalence of depression. Multiple studies have noted that the risk of suicide is related to the following factors: depressive episode severity, psychiatric comorbidities such as anxiety or substance use disorders, poor health status, and loss of functionality. There is a significant overlap between the symptoms of depression and medical illnesses. These symptoms are often nonspecific, such as loss of energy or appetite, insomnia, and somatic complaints. Suicidal behavior in depressed patients is associated with reduced social support and loneliness. Approximately 75% of patients that committed suicide were evaluated by their primary care provider within the previous 30 days, and about 33% within the previous week. It is therefore imperative that depression screenings be performed regularly with a validated tool to address confounding factors in this age group. The Cornell Scale for Depression in Dementia or the five-item Geriatric Depression Scale (**Table 2**) are such tools. The Cornell Scale for Depression in Dementia (CSDD) has a sensitivity of 93% and a specificity of 97% and is a 19-item screening tool that can be used in older patients (**Table 3**). It retains its validity when used in patients with dementia and has questions related to mood, behavior, physical signs, cyclic functions, and ideational disturbances.[12] It takes approximately 30 minutes to administer and can be performed by physicians or nursing staff. The Geriatric Depression Scale (GDS) is a self-report questionnaire and comes in several different forms and lengths including a four, five, 15, and 30-question question design (GDS-4, GDS-5, GDS-5, GDS-30), all of which are designed to screen for depression in the elderly (**Table 4**). The GDS 30 and GDS 15 are the most reliable with a sensitivity of 94% and specificity of 81%, but do not perform well in patients with underlying dementia.[11,13]

Pharmacotherapy with selective serotonin reuptake inhibitors (SSRIs) remain the treatment of choice for the geriatric patient with depression. Pharmaceutical intervention requires thoughtful selection given the pharmacokinetic changes in the elderly combined with the potential for adverse drug interaction due to polypharmacy in this population. **Table 5** summarizes the salient features to aid in distinguishing among delirium, dementia, and/or depression.

Elder Abuse

Elder abuse and neglect take many forms including physical abuse, psychological abuse, caregiver neglect, self-neglect, and even financial exploitation. Unfortunately, elder abuse is still significantly underreported with estimates in the United States of over 2 million geriatric patients per year. Cognitive and functional impairment are contributors to the underreported rate. Vigilance is paramount for its discovery while evaluating patients in the ED, paying close attention to those patients presenting with unexplained injuries or those in various stages of healing. If suspected, the patient should not be allowed to return to the potentially abusive environment and Adult Protective Services should be notified.

Emergency Department Evaluation

Establish the patient's baseline

When evaluating the geriatric patient with psychiatric symptoms in the ED it is important to consider the unique aspects of this patient population. As discussed, there is a high prevalence of baseline cognitive deficits in geriatric patients which may limit their ability to provide a comprehensive history. As such, every effort should be made to obtain a comprehensive history from both the patient and the patient's caregivers or

Table 2	
Five item geriatric depression scale[11]	
Choose the Best Answer for How You Have Felt Over the Past week:	
Are you basically satisfied with your life?	Yes/**No**
Do you often get bored?	**Yes**/No
Do you often feel helpless?	**Yes**/No
Do you prefer to stay at home rather than going out and doing new things?	**Yes**/No
Do you feel pretty worthless the way you are now?	**Yes**/No

Scoring: Bolded answers receive 1 point. A score of 2 or more is considered a positive result.

Table 3
Cornell scale for depression in dementia[12]

A. Mood-Related Signs

1	Anxiety (anxious expression, ruminations, worrying)	a 0 1 2
2	Sadness (sad expression, sad voice, tearfulness)	a 0 1 2
3	Lack of reactivity to pleasant events	a 0 1 2
4	Irritability (easily annoyed, short tempered)	a 0 1 2

B. Behavioral Disturbances

5	Agitation (restlessness, handwringing, hairpulling)	a 0 1 2
6	Retardation (slow movements, slow speech, slow reactions)	a 0 1 2
7	Multiple Physical Complaints (score 0 if GI symptoms only)	a 0 1 2
8	Loss of interest, less involved in usual activities (score only if change occurred acutely – less than 1 month)	a 0 1 2

C. Physical Signs

9	Appetite loss (eating less than usual)	a 0 1 2
10	Weight Loss (score 2 if greater than 5 lbs in 1 month)	a 0 1 2
11	Lack of energy (fatigues easily, unable to sustain activities) (score only if change occurred acutely – less than 1 month)	a 0 1 2

D. Cyclic Functions

12	Diurnal variation on mood (symptoms worse in the morning)	a 0 1 2
13	Difficulty falling asleep (later than usual for this person)	a 0 1 2
14	Multiple awakenings during sleep	a 0 1 2
15	Early morning awakening (earlier than usual for this person)	a 0 1 2

E. Ideational Disturbances

16	Suicide (feels life is not worth living, has suicidal wishes, or makes suicide attempt)	a 0 1 2
17	Poor self-esteem (self-blame, self-depreciation, feelings of failure)	a 0 1 2
18	Pessimism (anticipation of the worst)	a 0 1 2
19	Mood-congruent delusions (delusions of poverty, illness, or loss)	a 0 1 2

Total Score
>10 probably major depressive episode, >18 definite major depressive episode.
Scoring System: a = unable to evaluate 0 = absent, 1 = mild or intermittent, 2 = severe.
Ratings should be based on symptoms and signs occurring during the week prior No score should be given if symptoms result from physical disability or illness.

other relevant persons. For instance, it may be necessary to speak with family or caregivers arriving with the patient in the emergency department. Speaking with family, caregivers, or nursing or other facility staff over the phone may also facilitate a good patient history. Every effort should be made to *obtain a baseline mental status and level of function*, which may include questions regarding the patient's baseline activities of daily living (ADLs) and ambulatory status.[6] Obtaining and reviewing records from the Electronic Medical Records (EMR), other health care facilities, or nursing facilities may be helpful in addition to speaking with the patient's Primary Care Provider (PCP). A thorough review of the patient's medical, surgical, social, and medication history should be conducted.

Medication Review

Medication history is important in all populations but bears a special significance in the elderly. Special considerations of pharmacology in the geriatric age group

Table 4
15-Item geriatric depression scale[11]

Choose the Best Answer for How You Have Felt Over the Past Week:	
Are you basically satisfied with your life?	Yes/**No**
Have you dropped many of your activities and interests?	**Yes**/No
Do you feel that your life is empty?	**Yes**/No
Do you often get bored?	**Yes**/No
Are you in good spirits most of the time?	Yes/**No**
Are you afraid that something bad is going to happen to you?	**Yes**/No
Do you feel happy most of the time?	Yes/**No**
Do you often feel hopeless?	**Yes**/No
Do you prefer to stay at home, rather than going out and doing new things?	**Yes**/No
Do you feel you have more problems with memory than most?	**Yes**/No
Do you feel it is wonderful to be alive now?	Yes/**No**
Do you feel pretty worthless the way you are now?	**Yes**/No
Do you feel full of energy?	Yes/**No**
Do you feel that your situation is hopeless?	**Yes**/No
Do you think that most people are better off than you are?	**Yes**/No

Scoring: Bolded answers receive 1 point. A score of more than 5 suggests depression that should be further evaluated clinically.

include altered physiology and pharmacokinetics. These changes should significantly alter management styles and need to be at the forefront of decision-making when treating a geriatric patient so that the most appropriate and safe intervention may be selected. Given that 58% of geriatric patients take more than 5 medications daily (with 18% of this group taking more than 10), polypharmacy puts this group at increased risk for drug-drug interactions.[1] Adverse drug reactions are common iatrogenic causes of altered mental status and psychiatric symptoms in the elderly. Older patients experience physiologic changes that may cause abnormalities in the way certain medications are metabolized or distributed. For instance, the number of hepatocytes wanes and liver enzyme activity decreases with age, meaning that medications that rely on hepatic metabolism may be metabolized more slowly.[15] Similarly, older patients experience decreased glomerular filtration rates (GFR) and are more susceptible to nephrotoxicity.[15] The body's composition also changes; older patients tend to have a higher percentage of body fat vs. water or lean mass compared to younger patients.[15] **Table 6** lists some of the common physiologic and pharmacokinetic changes that occur with the aging process and how those changes may affect total body drug levels and metabolism. A drug's solubility may affect its distribution and thus affect the body. The American Geriatric Society's Updated Beer's Criteria for Potentially Inappropriate Medication Use in Older Adults is a helpful reference tool that may assist the emergency physician to determine whether a medication is appropriate for the elderly patient–and whether a particular medication may be contributing to the patient's acute symptoms. For instance, a physician may consult Beer's criteria and realize that a patient's psychiatric symptoms may be secondary to tramadol-induced hyponatremia from iatrogenic SIADH.[16] The list continues to be updated by the American Geriatrics Society, with the last update in 2019 containing a review of current literature from an interdisciplinary expert panel.[17]

Table 5
The features of dementia, delirium, and depression[14]

	Delirium	Dementia	Depression
Onset	Acute or subacute (hours or days)	Gradual over years Insidious in nature	Over days or weeks May coincide with life changes
Orientation	Fluctuating the impairment of sense of time, place and person	Increasingly impaired sense of time and place	Normal
Thoughts	Bizarre and vivid thoughts Frightening thoughts and ideas Paranoid thoughts	Repetitiveness of thought Reduced interests Difficulty making logical connections Slow processing of thought	Slowed thought processes Preoccupied by sadness and hopelessness Negative thoughts about self Reduced interest
Memory and Cognition	Immediate memory impaired Attention and concentration impaired	Impaired recent memory As progresses, long-term memory affected Associated cognitive deficits such as word finding, judgement and abstract thinking	Recent memory sometimes impaired Long-term memory intact Patchy memory loss Poor attention
Duration	Usually brief lasting hours to days	Months or years and usually progressive	At least 2 weeks (but can be months or years)
Daily Course	Fluctuates, worse at night or in the dark May have lucid periods	Variable depending on type	Worse in the morning with improvement as day progresses
Alertness	Fluctuates-lethargic or hypervigilant	Normal	Normal
Sleep	Confusion disturbs sleep (reverse sleep-wake cycle) Nocturnal confusion Vivid and disturbing nightmares	Disturbed 24-hour clock mechanism	Early morning waking or intermittent sleeping patterns
Other	May be a consequence of drug interaction or reaction, physical disease, psychological issue or environmental change	May be able to conceal or compensate for deficits (early)	Often masked May or may not have past history

Table 6 Physiologic and pharmacokinetic changes with normal aging	
Physiology/Pharmacokinetic Changes	**Effects**
Decreased albumin	Increased concentration of drug
Decreased GFR	Medication accumulation
Reduced hepatic blood flow	Medication accumulation
Increased body fat	Increased half-life of lipid-soluble drugs
Reduced dopamine and cholinergic function	Increased sensitivity to extrapyramidal symptoms and anticholinergic medications
Reduced total body water	Vulnerable to medication toxicity

Delirium Screen

The emergency physician should employ several screening examinations to assess for the presence of delirium in elderly patients. A delirium triage screen (DTS), as shown in **Fig. 1**,[1,18] is sensitive for the identification of delirium in the ED and may help the clinician identify a delirious patient.[1,18] The DTS can be administered in less than 20 seconds and has a sensitivity of 98% when performed by non-physicians and physicians making it an ideal rapid rule out delirium triage tool. There are 2 components to the DTS. The first is altered level of consciousness assessed by observing the patient and scoring them on the Richmond Agitation Sedation Scale (RASS **Table 7**). The second component is inattention tested by having the patient spell the word LUNCH backwards. If the patient's level of consciousness is normal AND they make zero or only one error spelling LUNCH backwards then the DTS is negative and delirium has been ruled out.

If the patient has an altered level of consciousness or makes 2 or more errors spelling the word LUNCH backwards then the DTS is positive. A separate, more specific delirium assessment such as the Brief Confusion Assessment Method (bCAM) is needed for delirium validation. The bCAM has four features that include (1) altered

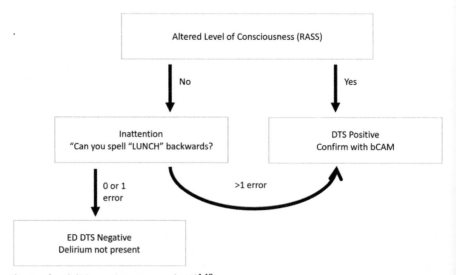

Fig. 1. The delirium triage screen (DTS)[1,18].

Table 7
Richmond agitation sedation scale (RASS)

RASS	Description
+4	Overly combative, violent, immediate danger to self
+3	Very agitated, pulls or removes tubes, catheters; aggressive
+2	Agitated, frequent and non-purposeful movement
+1	Restless, anxious but movements not aggressive or vigorous
0	Alert and calm
−1	Mildly drowsy, not fully alert, but has sustained awakening (>10 seconds)
−2	Moderate drowsy, briefly awakens with eye contact to voice (<10 seconds)
−3	Very drowsy, movement or eye opening to voice but no eye contact
−4	No response to voice, but movement or eye opening to physical stimulation
−5	No response to voice or physical stimulation

A patient with a RASS of −1 or +1 can have a subtle presentation.

mental status, (2) inattention, (3) altered level of consciousness (LOC), and disorganized thinking. The bCAM assessment can be completed in less than two minutes and has a sensitivity of 84% and a specificity of 96%.[1,18]

Evaluation

After a thorough history has been obtained and the patient has been screened for delirium, it is important to conduct a thorough physical examination. Psychiatric chief complaints may be the manifestation of many organic illnesses and the physical examination is a key component of diagnosis; especially in a patient unable to provide a first-hand history. Vital signs should also be obtained, including a core temperature and oxygen saturation.

The physical examination should include complete exposure of the patient, including examining the patient's back, genitalia, and extremities for signs of infection, neglect, or abuse[6] (for instance, a patient with altered mental status and diabetes may be unable to articulate scrotal pain, and a case of Fournier's gangrene may be missed if the patient is not properly exposed). Signs of trauma including bruises, occipital hematoma, or areas of tenderness should be noted, and the patient presenting with psychiatric symptoms should receive a full neurologic examination.[6] The American College of Emergency Physicians (ACEP) has created a bedside tool titled "ADEPT" that may be used in practice to assist in the evaluation of the confused geriatric patient.[6]

Assessment

A thorough workup should be initiated, as the differential diagnosis of altered mental status or psychiatric complaints in the elderly population is broad. Some common causes include infection, vitamin deficiencies, trauma, intracranial hemorrhage, malignancy, stroke, hypoxia, acute coronary syndrome, metabolic conditions such as hepatic encephalopathy, thyroid disturbances, diabetic emergencies, or iatrogenic causes like medication-adverse drug reactions, A point-of-care glucose check should always be performed in geriatric psychiatric patients. A complete blood count, complete metabolic panel, urinalysis, and an EKG are a typical part of the ED workup for a geriatric patient with altered mental status.[19] Computed tomography (CT) images of the patient's head, troponin testing, blood cultures, and other more specific, targeted

| Table 8 |
| Common laboratory and imaging evaluation for the geriatric patient[1,6,9] |

Generally Applicable	CBC with Differential, CMP, EKG, POC Glucose, CXR
Infection	Urinalysis, urine culture, blood cultures, lactate, CXR, head, chest or abdominal CT, bladder scan, lumbar puncture
Acute Coronary Syndrome/Cardiac Etiology	Troponin, BNP (Brain Natriuretic Peptide), CXR
Ischemic Stroke	Head CT, CT angiography, CT Perfusion, MRI (Magnetic Resonance Imaging)
Metabolic and Toxicology	VBG or ABG (Arterial Blood Gas), carboxyhemoglobin, toxicology screen, drug levels, alcohol level, TSH/free T4, POC glucose
Trauma	CT head, chest, abdomen/pelvis, PT/INR, PTT if anticoagulated

tests may be necessary on a case-by-case basis to help narrow the diagnosis. See **Table 8** for common laboratory and imaging tests. Of note, this list is not comprehensive but is a starting point to supplement clinical acumen. Clinicians should formulate comprehensive differential diagnoses and workups using their clinical judgment.

Management

During the evaluation, the safety of the patient and emergency department staff is equally as important as treating the underlying etiology of the patient's delirium. Factors that may agitate the patient such as pain, nausea, urinary or bowel retention, or dehydration should be addressed as doing so may aid in preventing or reducing the severity of delirium.[6]

First-line delirium treatment includes addressing these factors and employing comfort and screening measures that may be introduced system-wide to minimize geriatric patients' risk of delirium. These include keeping the patient's stay in the ED and hospital as close to their familiar environment as possible and minimizing restrictions on the patient's mobility. Use Foley catheters, IV tubing, blood pressure cuffs, monitor leads, and bed alarms only when necessary for the patient's treatment or safety.[6] The ED environment should be as calm and orienting as possible. Avoid placing patients in hallway beds, keep clocks visible, minimize noise, and ensure that the patient has their glasses and hearing aids.[1,6] Keep the room well-lit during the day and provide visual access to windows if possible.[1,20] Allow the patient easy access to toileting, walking aids, and sustenance if it is safe to do so.[6] Familiar faces and personal care can help to prevent and treat delirium. Family, caregivers, or other support persons should be encouraged to remain at the bedside and to bring other reminders of a familiar environment, if possible.[1] If this is not possible, a sitter may help the patient with re-orientation.

If these interventions are unsuccessful and/or the patient displays behavior that presents a potential safety hazard to themselves or others, verbal de-escalation techniques should be attempted as the next step. ACEP's ADEPT Tool provides a list of key points for verbal de-escalation with the geriatric patient as listed in **Box 1**.[6]

Chemical and physical restraints should be the absolute last remaining options with the geriatric patient and only be utilized after all other methods to calm and redirect the patient have been unsuccessful or impossible. If the patient's behavior presents an immediate threat to the safety of themselves or the staff, immediate chemical intervention and/or physical restraint is needed.

Box 1
Verbal De-Escalation Principles

- Respect personal space
- Do not be provocative
- Establish verbal contact
- Be concise and use simple language
- Identify the patient's wants and feelings
- Listen closely to what the patient is saying
- Agree or agree to disagree
- Set clear limits
- Offer choices and optimism
- Debrief the patient and staff

Link[6]: https://www.acep.org/adept/.

Table 9
Medications for the treatment of acute delirium in the ED geriatric patient

Route	Medication	Dose	Adverse Drug Reactions
PO (ODT or SL)	Haloperidol	0.25–0.5 mg q1h, max 3–5 mg/24 hours	Orthostatic hypotension, somnolence, QT prolongation, dystonia, contraindicated in Parkinson's
	Olanzapine	2.5–5 mg BID PRN	Orthostatic hypotension, somnolence
Quetiapine	12.5–25 mg BID PRN	Orthostatic hypotension, somnolence	
Risperidone	0.5 mg BID max 6mg/24 hours, orthostatic hypotension	dystonia/EP side effects	avoid in dementia
IM	Haloperidol	0.5–1 mg IM q1 hr, max 3–5 mg/24 hrs (avoid≥5 mg doses)	Orthostatic hypotension, somnolence, QT prolongation, dystonia/EP side effects, contraindicated in Parkinson's
	Olanzapine	2.5–5 mg BID PRN	Orthostatic hypotension, somnolence
	Ziprasidone	10 mg q2h PRN, max 40 mg/24 hrs	Orthostatic hypotension, somnolence, caution in uncontrolled CHF or cardiac disease
IV	Haloperidol	0.25–1 mg IV	IM is preferred over IV because of increased risk for extrapyramidal side effects, orthostatic hypotension, and QT prolongation/torsade. Administer IV in a monitored setting.

Adapted from ACEP's ADEPT Tool[6,19,21]

> **Box 2**
> **Approach to the elderly patient with psychiatric symptoms in the ED**
>
> - Screen for depression, delirium, and elder abuse
> - Take a thorough history, including medication reconciliation, baseline cognitive and functional status
> - Perform a thorough physical examination, including full skin and GU examination
> - Perform a thorough workup for organic causes of the patient's symptoms
> - Minimize the patient's discomfort including nausea, urinary retention, and other factors
> - Provide access to mobility assistive devices, hearing devices, clocks, windows, and familiar faces.
> - Use verbal de-escalation if possible
> - If medication is needed, use oral medications first or choose a medication that the patient is already taking
> - If oral medication is not an option, use the lowest dose possible of IM or IV medications

Physical restraints may be needed to prevent the patient from harming himself or herself and others. Types of physical restraints include (but are not limited to) soft wrist/ankle restraints, straps or belts for chairs or wheelchairs, mitt restraints, and wheelchair safety bars. Bed side rails may be considered physical restraints if a patient cannot remove themselves from the bed due to these physical barriers. If a patient requires physical restraint, every effort should be made to ensure this is done safely. A patient in four-point restraints should never be immobilized in the prone position as this may lead to suffocation. When employing four-point immobilization, 5 team members should ideally be present; one for each limb and one to manage the team. Immobilization for a prolonged period may lead to rhabdomyolysis, a potentially fatal condition. Physical restraints should be used for the minimal amount of time required and should be removed when it is safe to do so, and the least-restricting physical restraint sufficient for safety should be used.

Regarding chemical restraint, if possible, it is best to start with oral medications. If the patient is on an antipsychotic as a regularly prescribed medication, it may be best to administer an additional dose of that medication. If the patient is not typically on antipsychotic medications there are several oral options: Risperidone, Olanzapine, Haloperidol, and Quetiapine.[21–24] If giving PO medications is impossible, or the medications administered are ineffective, the use of IM or IV medications is the next option and includes the following: Ziprasidone, Olanzapine, and Haloperidol. When administering medications to the geriatric population, physicians should follow the "lowest dose" rule, meaning that they should use the lowest dose of medication possible for patient safety. **Table 9** outlines the recommended dosing for the ED geriatric patient as adapted from ACEP's ADEPT Tool. Physical restraints may be a necessary addition to medications in order to keep the patients and staff safe. One study demonstrated that elderly patients placed in physical restraints in the ED most often have a medically necessary reason. Over 57%, of patients requiring physical restraints were from nursing homes and over one-third of these patients had a serious medical illness requiring ICU admission. The overwhelming majority, more than 92% of patients, required two-point soft restraints. There were no major or minor adverse physical outcomes.[25]

It is worth noting that antipsychotics have a black-box warning from the Food and Drug Administration (FDA) for increased mortality in the elderly with dementia-related psychosis.[6,19] Additionally, medications that are typically used for younger patients such as benzodiazepines and diphenhydramine are not recommended for elderly patients secondary to their adverse drug reactions in this age group. Benzodiazepines, if they absolutely must be used, should be administered in a much smaller dose than for younger patients (unless continuing home medication dose to avoid withdrawal or treating acute alcohol withdrawal).[21] Physical restraints should also be avoided and used only as a temporary, last resort due to the risk of injury, psychological distress, and metabolic disturbances.

The disposition of a patient with an acute psychiatric emergency is challenging. Any patient with an acute change in mental status should be admitted to the inpatient setting. Criteria for discharge include an identified, reversible, easily addressed underlying cause, improving clinical status, and adequate home support including adequate supervision, care, and assistance with ADLs at home.[21]

SUMMARY

The diagnosis of an acute psychiatric emergency in the geriatric patient who presents to the ED remains a diagnostic and management challenge particularly when these conditions often overlap and coexist. Failure to recognize elder psychiatric problems carries a significantly increased morbidity for the patient. It is therefore paramount that ED clinicians can not only diagnose delirium, depression, and/or elder abuse in the geriatric population but also manage these patients appropriately and in a timely fashion to improve outcomes. **Box 2** should serve as a guide when you encounter your next elderly patient in the ED with psychiatric symptoms.

CLINICS CARE POINTS

- Delirium is an acute change in attention and awareness, while dementia is a process that develops over time without affecting attention and consciousness, and tends not to fluctuate acutely

- Altered mental status and psychiatric symptoms are common manifestations of organic processes; new psychiatric diagnoses causing psychosis are rare in the elderly population

- Remember to screen geriatric patients for depression, delirium, and elder abuse with validated screening tools

- Establishing a patient's functional baseline (including ADLs and baseline cognition) and performing a thorough medication reconciliation are essential components of the emergency evaluation of the geriatric patient

- First-line treatment and prevention of delirium include addressing pain, nausea, urinary or bowel retention, dehydration, and other factors that may cause discomfort; as well as keeping noise, alarms, and other disturbances to a minimum. Maintenance of mobility, hearing aids, and other assistive devices, and familiar visitors to the patient's bedside can also help minimize delirium.

- If chemical restraints are needed, start with a medication the patient is already taking, and use oral medications if possible

- If oral medication is not an option, Ziprasidone, Olanzapine, and Haloperidol are options; give at the lowest dose possible.

DISCLOSURE

The authors have nothing to disclose.

REFERENCES

1. Emergency Geriatric, Department guidelines. (n.d.), ACEP.org. https://www.acep.org/patient-care/policy-statements/geriatric-emergency-department-guidelines/.
2. One in 10 older Americans has dementia. (2022, October 22). ScienceDaily. https://www.sciencedaily.com/releases/2022/10/221024131046.htm.
3. Han JH, Zimmerman EE, Cutler N, et al. Delirium in older emergency department patients: recognition, risk factors, and psychomotor subtypes. Acad Emerg Med 2009;16(3):193–200.
4. Quirk S, Pettett V. Rationale for change, . *Diagnostic and Statistical Manual of Mental Disorders*. 5th ed.. https://doi.org/10.4324/9780429325694-4.
5. Rossom R., Anderson P., Greer N., Delirium : Screening , Prevention , and Diagnosis – A Systematic Review of the Evidence. Evidence-based Synth Progr Cent. Published online 2011:1-91. Available at: http://www.ncbi.nlm.nih.gov/pubmed/22206108. Accessed December 23, 2022.
6. Shenvi C., Kennedy M., Wilson M.P., et al., ADEPT: Confusion and Agitation in the Elderly ED Patient. ACEP. Published 2022. Available at: https://www.acep.org/patient-care/adept/. Accessed December 23, 2022.
7. American Geriatrics Society. Clinical Practice Guideline for Postoperative Delirium in Older Adults.; 2014. Available at: file:///C:/Users/monic/Downloads/AGS_PostOp_Delirium_Final_pdf. Accessed December 23, 2022.
8. Oldham MA, Flanagan NM, Khan A, et al. Responding to ten common delirium misconceptions with best evidence: an educational review for clinicians. J Neuropsychiatry Clin Neurosci 2018;30(1):51–7.
9. Karlsson S, Bucht G, Sandman PO. Physical restraints in geriatric care. Scand J Caring Sci 1998;12:48–56.
10. Obuobi-Donkor G, Nkire N, Agyapong VIO. Prevalence of major depressive disorder and correlates of thoughts of death, suicidal behaviour, and death by suicide in the geriatric population—a general review of literature. Behav Sci 2021; 11(11). https://doi.org/10.3390/bs11110142.
11. Maurer DM, Raymond TJ, Davis BN. Depression: screening and diagnosis. Am Fam Physician 2018;98(8):508–15.
12. Alexopoulos G, Abrams R, Young R, et al. Cornell scale for depression in dementia. Biol Psychiatry 1998;23:271–84.
13. Yesavage JA, Brink T, Rose T, et al. Development and validation of a geriatric depression screening scale: a preliminary report. J Psychiatry Res 1983;17:37–49. Available at: http://web.stanford.edu/~yesavage/GDS.english.long.html.
14. Queensland Mind Essentials. Caring for a Person with Dementia. Published online 2006. Available at: https://www.health.qld.gov.au/__data/assets/pdf_file/0023/444524/dementia.pdf. Accessed December 23, 2022.
15. Melady D. Medication Management in the Older ED Patient: Physiology of Aging. Geri-EM. Published 2013. Available at: https://geri-em.com/medication-management/physiology-of-aging/2019 American Geriatrics Society Beers Criteria® Update Expert Panel. Accessed December 23, 2022.
16. Croke L. Beers criteria for inappropriate medication use in older patients: an update from the AGS. Am Fam Physician 2020;101(1):56–7.
17. By the 2019 American Geriatrics Society Beers Criteria® Update Expert Panel. American Geriatrics Society 2019 Updated AGS Beers Criteria® for Potentially Inappropriate Medication Use in Older Adults. J Am Geriatr Soc 2019;67(4):674–94. https://doi.org/10.1111/jgs.15767.

18. Han JH, Wilson A, Vasilevskis EE, et al. Diagnosing delirium in older emergency department patients: Validity and reliability of the delirium triage screen and the brief confusion assessment method. Ann Emerg Med 2013;62(5):457–65.
19. Inouye SK, Baker S, Erickson K. et al., Delirium in the Older Emergency Department Patient (ED-DEL) Change Package and Toolkit. Published online 2020. Available at: https://s8637.pcdn.co/wp-content/uploads/2021/04/ED_Delirium_Toolkit_4.28.21.pdf. Accessed December 23, 2022.
20. Lee HJ, Bae E, Lee HY, et al. Association of natural light exposure and delirium according to the presence or absence of windows in the intensive care unit. Acute Crit Care 2021;36(4):332–41.
21. Shenvi C, Kennedy M, Austin CA, et al. Managing delirium and agitation in the older emergency department patient: the ADEPT tool. Ann Emerg Med 2020; 75(2):136–45.
22. Borja B, Borja CS, Gade S. Psychiatric emergencies in the geriatric population. Clin Geriatr Med 2007;23(2):391–vii.
23. Sikka V, Kalra S, Galwankar S. Psychiatric emergencies in the elderly. Emerg Med Clin North Am 2015;33(4):825–39, published correction appears in Emerg Med Clin North Am. 2016 Feb;34(1):xv. Sagar, Galwankar [corrected to Galwankar, Sagar].
24. Antai-Otong D. Managing geriatric psychiatric emergencies: delirium and dementia. Nurs Clin North Am 2003;38(1):123–35.
25. Swickhamer C, Colvig C, Chan SB. Restraint use in the elderly emergency department patient. J Emerg Med 2013;44(4):869–74.

Pediatric Psychiatric Emergencies

Purva Grover, MD, MBA[a],*, Manya Kumar, MBBS[b]

KEYWORDS

- Pediatric emergencies • Suicide • Homicidal ideation
- Acutely violent pediatric patients • Emergency department

KEY POINTS

- The number of pediatric psychiatric emergencies has risen in the last few years.
- Depression, anxiety, and behavioral challenges are the most common presentations.
- Pediatric psychiatric emergencies are difficult to diagnose because of variable presentation, but early diagnosis and treatment improves clinical outcome.
- Emphasis should be given on the de-escalation of the patient, age-appropriate interviewing, and ruling out organic pathologies.
- A multidisciplinary approach involving the child's primary care physician and psychiatrist should be adopted, keeping available resources in mind.

INTRODUCTION

Pediatric psychiatric emergencies have been exponentially increasing in the last decade and especially so in last few years. In recent years, national surveys have shown major increases in mental health symptoms, including depressive symptoms and suicidal ideation in the pediatric and adolescent population. From 2009 to 2019,[1–3] the proportion of high school students reporting persistent feelings of sadness or hopelessness increased by 40%; those seriously considering suicide increased by 36%; and those with an actual suicide plan increased by 44%.[2,4] The COVID-19 pandemic has dramatically changed the milieu for these patients, including how they attend school, interact with friends, and receive health care. In the last 5 years, pediatric mental health–related visits to emergency department (ED) for depression, anxiety, and behavioral challenges have increased by over 45%.[3–5] This article explores the definition, scope, clinical presentation, and management of these

[a] Cleveland Clinic, 6780 Mayfield Road, Mayfield Heights, OH 44124, USA; [b] Vardhman Mahavir Medical College, Safdarjung Hospital, Ansari Nagar East, New Delhi, Delhi 110029, India
* Corresponding author. 39500 Patterson Lane, Solon, OH 44139.
E-mail address: groverp@ccf.org

Emerg Med Clin N Am 42 (2024) 151–162
https://doi.org/10.1016/j.emc.2023.06.017
0733-8627/24/© 2023 Elsevier Inc. All rights reserved.

situations in the emergency setting. It discusses both pharmacologic and nonpharmacologic treatment stabilization options.

CASE VIGNETTE

Nine-year-old AJ was in a quiet room at his school counselor's office after he got into a fight with some other schoolmates. She noticed superficial cuts on his right wrist. When she asked about them, he became agitated, pacing in the room. All attempts to calm him failed, and he started throwing things around in the room and hitting his head on the table. Emergency medical services (EMS) was called for transport to the ED. Enroute, he continued to say that he wanted to kill himself and banged his head into the windows. This caused his forehead to bleed. When staff attempted first aid, he attacked them, scratching one of them in the face. He was then placed into 4-point leather restraints and transported to your ED, where he is now growling and spitting at you and the ED staff. He is tachycardic and tachypneic. Blood pressure could not be obtained because he is thrashing about. Your staff is apprehensive, and the parents at the bedside are extremely anxious.

MENTAL ILLNESS IN CHILDREN AND ADOLESCENTS

ED health care professionals often care for patients with previously diagnosed psychiatric illnesses who are ill, injured, or having a behavioral crisis. They also must identify and manage patients with previously undiagnosed and/or undetected conditions such as suicidal ideation, depression, anxiety, psychosis, substance use and abuse, and posttraumatic stress disorder. Mental health conditions now account for 10%-15% of ED visits by children and adolescents in the United States.[1] Treatment costs for pediatric mental health conditions are estimated to be $13 billion annually, surpassing the costs for asthma and all childhood infectious diseases combined. Many of these conditions have some form of prodromal features that may begin even earlier in life and often are difficult to detect. It is estimated that 50% to 70% of patients with mental health conditions do not receive treatment from a mental health professional; therefore, the ED has become the safety net for this population in times of crisis.[2] More than half of young patients who present to the ED with a new mental health condition have not previously been evaluated by an outpatient provider for psychiatric needs.[4] Earlier treatment has been shown to improve outcomes in first-episode psychosis, major depressive disorder (MDD), bipolar disorder, panic disorder, generalized anxiety disorder, and obsessive-compulsive disorder, highlighting the importance for ED providers to recognize psychiatric symptoms. One-half of all mental health visits are repeat visits, suggesting a lack of adequate care and follow-up.[3] One study found that the median wait time for an appointment with a child and adolescent psychiatrist was 50 days, and a recent study published in 2020 found that almost 10% of patients never established outpatient care.[5]

The increase in mental health–related visits disproportionately affects minority children, with a recent study conducted from 2012 to 2016 showing that Black and Hispanic children experienced higher rates of ED visits than non-Hispanic white children.[6] Studies show that Black and Hispanic children have lower medical expenditures, have fewer outpatient visits, and receive fewer medication prescriptions than white children and, thus, may use the ED as their primary source of medical care. The lack of outpatient care among minority children and psychosocial stressors likely are contributors to their increased use of the ED for mental health conditions.

Not only is the proportion of children and adolescents seen in the ED with mental health conditions increasing, but their average length of stay (LOS) also has become longer. Those with inpatient dispositions had an increased LOS, while those being discharged had a stable LOS, suggesting a delay not in ED provider decision-making, but rather delays with patient placement. One factor that may contribute to this delay is that inpatient psychiatric beds have decreased since the mid-1960s. A survey done by the National Pediatric Readiness Project[7] revealed that less than half of hospitals are prepared with policies for children with mental health conditions, and, in rural areas, less than one-third have policies in place or mental health transfer agreements, leading to an increased LOS as hospitals scramble to find bed placement for these patients. Most children are seen in general EDs (not pediatric-specific), which have been shown to be less prepared to provide optimal pediatric care.[8] This highlights the need for ED providers across all hospital EDs to be familiar with the most common mental health presentations in the pediatric population to effectively engage with and provide proper care and disposition to this at-risk population.[9,10]

Suicide in the United States currently ranks as the fourth leading cause of death for 10- to 14-year-olds and the third leading cause of death for 15- to 19-year-olds, accounting for 11.3% of all deaths in the latter age group.[11,12] More than half of adolescents 13 to 19 years of age have suicidal thoughts, nearly 250,000 adolescents attempt suicide each year, and up to 10% of children attempt suicide sometime during their lives. Of great concern is the fact that, despite its increasing prevalence, the risk of suicidal behavior in many children and adolescents is often undetected. One study found that 83% of adolescent patients who had attempted suicide were not recognized as suicidal by their primary care physicians.[13]

Patients who need mental health care require more complex resources that are difficult to procure. In a 2006 study, Santiago and colleagues[14–16] reported that 210 patients with a median age of 14 years and requiring psychiatric evaluation spent a median of 5.7 hours in the ED. Hospital police monitored 51.9% of these patients, and 45 patients exhibited dangerous behaviors. Among children who frequently used mental health services in the ED, approximately 50% of them were seen again within 2 months of their initial visit, which suggests that patterns of return visits are high for psychiatric patients.[13,17,18] Repeat patients are more likely to threaten to harm others; to have a diagnosis of adjustment, conduct, or oppositional disorder; and to be under the care of a child welfare agency. Repeat users were also significantly more likely than one-time patients to be less compliant with outpatient follow-up, be admitted to the hospital, and require more social support. These youth also have increased risk of involvement with juvenile justice; a large proportion of them have related behavioral, emotional, and cognitive disabilities and have greater difficulty remaining in residential treatment.[15] The total proportion of children admitted to general inpatient services from the ED for mental health problems is also increasing.[19]

Common types of psychiatric emergencies include suicidal threats or behavior, assaultive, destructive, otherwise violent behavior, and acute mental status changes (intoxication, agitation, psychosis, delirium, or extreme anxiety with physical symptoms) when a medical ideology has not been excluded.

GENERAL PRINCIPLES

The ED highlights the crucial role that safety plays in the psychiatric evaluation in youth. The use of quiet rooms, continuous one-on-one observation, medications for agitation, and physical restraints are at times necessary to contain patients who pose an eminent threat to themselves or others. Simple measures to address both physical and emotional safety may help avoid the need for more restrictive and/or invasive measures later in the evaluation and treatment processes. Obtaining collateral information is a mandatory component of every evaluation. Children who are struggling are often unable to volunteer information or reach out for help. They also may not be in an emotional or developmental level such that they can articulate the thought processes well. It is crucial, particularly in emergencies, to clarify and obtain collateral information from the patient's family, siblings, counselors, and teachers, as appropriate, in the clinical setting. Psychiatric evaluation of children and teenagers requires a deep understanding of cognitive, emotional, and physical development. Personalizing the interview questions and tailoring the strategy to the patient's age and developmental status is crucial for gaining trust, gathering information, and also being able to partner with the patient in determining a plan of care.

The prevalence of coexisting medical illness in psychiatric patients has been reported to be as high as 50%. An untreated medical illness often causes deterioration of baseline cognitive function in patients with a known psychiatric disorder. The prevalence of medical disease in patients seen in the ED with an acute exacerbation of an existing mental illness may be as high as 80%.[20] Up to 50% of patients demonstrate a causal relationship between acute medical and psychiatric complaints.

MEDICAL ASSESSMENT
The Medical Assessment Must Include Thoughtful Consideration to the Following Components

1. Is the patient stable or unstable?
2. Is the behavior the result of an underlying medical illness?
3. What is the severity of the primary mental disorder?
4. Is psychiatric consultation necessary?
5. Does the patient need to be detained to facilitate emergency treatment?
6. What capability does the psychiatric facility have to treat medical conditions?

The standard workup should include a thorough history, focused physical examination, and vital sign assessment. For children and teens, the history should concentrate on the precipitant of the mental health crisis. Particular areas to review include school performance, relationship with family and peers, living situation, family composition, sexuality, and neighborhood environment. Look for abrasions or contusions that may represent recent trauma or unsuspected head injury. Identify subtle, focal weakness or neglect suggestive of possible neurologic impairment. The patient's vital signs should be scrutinized for evidence of shock, metabolic derangement, or infection. Routine lab work for "medical clearance" has fallen out of favor for pediatric patients, but laboratory and imaging studies must be performed if there are any clinical concerns.[21–23]

SUICIDAL IDEATION/PLAN

Over the last few years, many strides have been made with the screening process for patients who present with suicidal ideation or thoughts. A comprehensive suicide risk assessment is necessary to categorize the patient's risk and appropriate level of care. Many suicide instruments utilized for this purpose include the Columbia suicide severity rating scale, Suicide Assessment Five step Evaluation and Triage (SAFE–TP), and the Ask Suicide Screening Questions (ASQ). The ED Screen for Teens At Risk of Suicide (ED-STARS) is one such multisite study, which successfully identified patient profiles for adolescents with elevated suicide risk.[24] The authors studied the association between these profiles and mental health service utilizations. Providers may use the screening tools while the patient is in triage to assign acuity levels and appropriate resources for patients.

One of the most important elements in caring for these patients is to determine the correct level of care and their final disposition. Patients of higher risk typically require inpatient admission. Safety planning and/or contracting for safety as a verbal or written record has been an effective tool. However, it is not contractual or binding in any way. In the document, clinicians, patients, and family can discuss warning signs, coping strategies, and safety net options. It is imperative to contact the patient's primary care physician, psychiatrist, and counselor as applicable for the patient to have a soft landing spot if they are discharged from the ED. Warm handoff in these cases can often prevent escalation and return visits to the ED. As most EDs are not equipped to have psychiatric assessment by psychiatrists or other professionals in the ED, the use of telepsychiatry has now become a viable option as appropriate for some of these patients. Innovative thinking in having a psychiatrist review the plan of care or even assess the patient while in the ED has shown to have high rate of success in the care of these patients. These are, unfortunately, resource-intensive situations, and often the emergency physician has to rely on the safety net outside the ED settings for appropriate care and follow-up.

HOMICIDAL IDEATION/AGGRESSION

Aggressive violent behavior can be a diagnosis unto itself but also may result from an underlying medical, toxicological, or mental problem, or a combination of these conditions. Symptoms can include restlessness, hyperactivity, confusion verbal threats, and frank violence toward property, others, or oneself. It is one of the most frequent causes of workplace injury violence. The basic strategies and priorities for evaluating the aggressive patient are similar to the ones detailed previously in the evaluation of the suicidal patient. The most important priority is always ensuring the safety of the patient and the ED staff. Verbal de-escalation, distraction techniques, and other behavior strategies have been shown to be effective in reducing the need for chemical or physical restraints. The presence or involvement of family members and other collaborative members of the patient's life can be calming to the patient; however, safety must always remain a top priority.

In the pediatric and adolescent patient population, restraints (either chemical and/or physical) can be very disturbing and can have long-lasting effects on the psyche and development. Patients with developmental, neurological, or language deficits are more prone to aggression since they cannot adequately communicate verbally. Appropriate understanding of the patient's developmental stage and social circumstance is important in their care. Because restraints have been associated with adverse outcomes, the Centers for Medicare and Medicaid and the Joint Commission have adopted regulations regarding appropriate use and monitoring of restraints.

The first step to treat acute agitation in the ED is de-escalation. Multiple agitation scales have been validated for ED use. The Behavior Activity Rating Scale[25] (**Table 1**) measures activity levels on a seven-point scale to determine the appropriate level of care needed. Richmond and colleagues[26] proposed a 10-point step model for de-escalation (**Table 2**).

If nonphysical de-escalation is ineffective, pharmacotherapy is indicated, with the goal being to calm rather than to completely sedate. Physicians should be aware of potential complications of pharmaceutical restraint, including cardiorespiratory and

Table 1 Behavioral activity rating scale (BARS)[25]	
1	Difficult or Unable to Arouse
2	Asleep but responds normally to verbal or physical contact
3	Drowsy, appears sedated
4	Quiet and awake (normal level of activity)
5	Signs of overt (physical or verbal) activity, calms down with instructions
6	Extremely or continuously active, not requiring restraint
7	Violent, requires restraint

central nervous system depression, extrapyramidal reaction, and QTC prolongation. Continuous cardiorespiratory monitoring is recommended (**Table 3**).

MAJOR DEPRESSIVE DISORDER

MDD is a psychiatric illness with a prevalence of about 5% to 8% prior to the age of 13 years.[27,28] It is defined as 2 or more weeks with feelings of sadness, plus 5 of the following symptoms: sleep disturbance, decreased interest, guilt, low energy, decreased concentration, decreased attention, psychomotor agitation or retardation, or suicidal ideation. Depression in the pediatric population can often present as irritability or more severe mood swings rather than sadness or anhedonia. The United States Preventative Services Task Force recommends routine screening for depression in adolescents older than 12 years. These patients often screen positive under routine questioning performed in ED triage. Those who screen positive for MDD must be linked with appropriate outpatient facilities, including intensive outpatient treatments, counseling, primary care, and psychiatry. An understanding of the local resources available in the community is extremely important for patient disposition. It is very rare for the ED to prescribe medications for new-onset diagnosis. However, some anxiolytics can be given on an as-needed basis after discussion with the patient's medical providers. Review appropriate coping skills and warning signs and ensure access to hotlines and other safety mechanisms.

ANXIETY

Anxiety disorders have a prevalence of 7% in youths aged 3 to 17 years and 35% in adolescents aged 13 to 18 years.[27,29] Common anxiety disorders in children and

Table 2 Ten domains of de-escalation, Richmond et al[26]	
1	Respect Personal Space
2	Do not be provocative
3	Establish verbal contact
4	Be concise
5	Identify wants and feelings
6	Listen closely to what the patient is saying
7	Agree or agree to disagree
8	Lay down the law and set clear limits
9	Offer choices and optimism
10	Debrief the patient and staff

Table 3
Medications

Class	Drug	Route	Dose	Onset of Action	Duration	Relative Contraindications	Side Effects	Comments
Anti-histaminic	Diphenhydramine	IM	0.5-1 mg/kg/dose (max 50 mg)		4–7 h	Prior paradoxical reaction to diphenhydramine, developmental delay, or current anticholinergic/ TCA use	QT prolongation	Consider early use Avoid use in delirium
		IV						
		PO	May repeat every 4–6 h	Peak onset ~ 1 to 2 h				
Benzo-diazepine	Lorazepam	IM	0.05 mg/kg (max 4 mc)	15–30 min		Disinhibition, respiratory inability	Respiratory depression, disinhibition	May be ineffective for acute delirium. If inadequate effect achieved after 2 doses or disinhibition occurs, consider addition of an antipsychotic
		IV	May repeat IV/IM every		60–120 min			
		PO	20 min or PO every 30 min	30–60 min				
	Midazolam	IV	0.3 mg/kg (max 5 mg) May repeat in 20 min		18–40 min			
Anti-psychotic	Olanzapine	ODT	If weight > 60 kg, 10 mg If weight 30–60 kg, 5 mg	15–30 min	30 h	QT prolongation, anticholinergic intoxication, active seizure disorder	QT prolongation, orthostatic hypotension	Consent < 4 years old IM olanzapine should not be given any sooner than 3 hours after lorazepam

(continued on next page)

Table 3
(continued)

Class	Drug	Route	Dose	Onset of Action	Duration	Relative Contraindications	Side Effects	Comments
	Risperidone	ODT	If weight 15–29 kg: 0.25 mg	Less than 60 min	15 h	QT prolongation, anticholinergic intoxication, active seizure disorder	QT prolongation, tachycardia, hypertension	Full effect may take 30 min. If IV ordered, EKG necessary prior to initiation
	Haloperidol	IM	0.025 mg/kg (max 5 mg)		3–6 h	QT prolongation, anticholinergic intoxication, active seizure disorder, withdrawal syndrome	QT prolongation, extra-pyramidal symptoms	
		IV	May repeat x 1 in 30 min					
Sedative/anesthetic	Ketamine	IM	2–4 mg/kg (max 200 mg)			Hypertensive urgency, increased ICP, phencyclidine poisoning	Tachycardia, hypertension	Obtain IV access and benzo-diazepines and/or antipsychotic medication. May be titrated on signs of lightening

adolescents include generalized anxiety disorder, panic disorder, social anxiety disorder, separation anxiety disorder, and phobias. Eating disorders are also prevalent in this age group, and anxiety plays a major role in management of these patients. Panic disorder is one of the most common presentations in the ED for noncardiac chest pain.

Generalized anxiety disorder is defined as excessive anxiety and worry that is difficult to control, present on more days than not for at least 6 months. This can cause significant distress and impede day-to-day functions in social and school settings. It is accompanied by restlessness, fatigability, difficulty with concentration, muscle tension, and sleep disturbance. Anxiety can be confused with attention deficit hyperactivity disorder (ADHD), but children with ADHD have difficulty with attention regardless of their anxiety level.

Patients with anxiety often can present with severe, vague somatic symptoms and might need an extensive medical workup if the diagnosis is not immediately clear or has not been established in the past. These youth are also at high risk of suicide attempts since anxiety and depression often coexist.

Panic disorders and panic attacks are frequently seen in the ED. Adolescents and young children can report a feeling of impending doom or intense fear or anxiety not accompanied by hyperventilation, resulting in paresthesias, shortness of breath, chest pain, and nausea. Panic attacks can be spontaneous, and sometimes no triggers can be identified. Because some of these panic attacks and anxiety attacks can closely mimic cardiogenic symptoms, it is extremely important to do a thorough medical examination, history, and appropriate testing before diagnosing the child with an anxiety disorder. A short-acting benzodiazepine can be used for treatment of an acute panic attack in the ED. Treatment of hyperventilation and coping skills are important to teach. Discuss these with the patient and family during assessment and management.

SUMMARY

Helping children to navigate the psychiatric crisis can put them on a path to recovery. Effective emergency evaluation and connection to care is essential. We need to continue to improve the capacity of our psychiatric emergency response system to battle this new public health crises. Treating children and adolescents in this context is a difficult task, made more so by the complexity of the child's symptoms, cognitive and emotional development, family complexity, and school and peer dynamics. In cases such as AJ's, several issues need to be addressed.

1. Immediate steps to deescalate patient
2. Ensuring safety of patient and staff taking care of him
3. Age-appropriate interview/evaluation of patient
4. Discussing and gathering secondary collaborating evidence (family, counsellors, and so on)
5. Determining safe disposition–discharge or admit
6. Connecting and understanding resources available in community for a safe landing spot.

CASE WRAP-UP

As the ED staff tries to deescalate AJ, his parents arrive at bedside. Mom shares that AJ usually responds better if he is in a quiet space where he is less stimulated and can pace around. In the meanwhile, the ED nurse has drawn up medications to be used for chemical restraint. You decide to hold off the medication, go inside the room and tell

AJ that you will dim the lights and leave him alone, so he feels better. It is a risk, but shared decision-making with family and ED staff makes it the next best decision. You continue to monitor AJ via camera, and within few minutes, he goes to lie on the cot and is visibly calmer. You re-enter the room with his family and establish rapport with AJ, who can establish trust and begin his healing process.

CLINICS CARE POINTS

- Mental health conditions account for 15% of ED visits by the pediatric population in the United States.
- They are often difficult to diagnose due to variable presentation from their adult counterparts.
- An early diagnosis and treatment can significantly affect the prognosis of several mental health conditions.
- Invest time in ED staff learning various nonpharmaceutical de-escalation strategies.
- Always consider medical organic reasons for the patients' presentation, even if they have an established diagnosis of a mental health pathology.
- In the ED, it is imperative that we address both the physical and emotional safety aspects of care.
- We need to determine the correct level of care of the patients according to the resources available at the level of the community.
- Working together with a psychiatrist or the patient's primary care physician and family is strongly recommended.

DISCLOSURE

The authors have nothing to disclose.

REFERENCES

1. Santillanes G, Axeen S, Lam CN, et al. National trends in mental health-related emergency department visits by children and adults, 2009-2015. Am J Emerg Med 2020;38:2536–44.
2. Hoffmann JA, Stack AM, Samnaliev M, et al. Trends in visits and costs for mental health emergencies in a pediatric emergency department, 2010-2016. Acad Pediatr 2019;19:386–93.
3. Soni A. Top Five Most Costly Conditions among Children, Ages 0-17, 2012: Estimates for the U.S. Civilian Noninstitutionalized Population. In: Statistical Brief (Medical Expenditure Panel Survey (US) [Internet]. Rockville (MD): Agency for Healthcare Research and Quality (US); 2015. 2001–. STATISTICAL BRIEF #472. PMID: 28783284.
4. Kalb LG, Stapp EK, Ballard ED, et al. Trends in psychiatric emergency department visits among youth and young adults in the U.S. Pediatrics 2019;143: e20182192.
5. World Health Organization. Improving the mental and brain health of children and adolescents. Available at: https://www.who.int/activities/Improving-the-mental-and-brain-health-ofchildren-and-adolescents.

6. Abrams AH, Badolato GM, Boyle MD, et al. Racial and ethnic disparities in pediatric mental health-related emergency department visits. Pediatr Emerg Care 2020. https://doi.org/10.1097/PEC.0000000000002221.

7. National pediatric readiness project-. JAMA Pediatr 2015;169(6):527–34.

8. Colizzi M, Lasalvia A, Ruggeri M. Prevention and early intervention in youth mental health: Is it time for a multidisciplinary and trans-diagnostic model for care? Int J Ment Health Syst 2020;14:23.

9. Fusar-Poli P. Integrated mental health services for the developmental period (0 to 25 years): a critical review of the evidence. Front Psychiatry 2019;10:355.

10. Stevens JR, Prince JB, Prager LM, et al. Psychotic disorders in children and adolescents: a primer on contemporary evaluation and management. Prim Care Companion CNS Disord 2014;16. PCC.13f01514.

11. Whitney DG, Peterson MDUS. national and state-level prevalence of mental health disorders and disparities of mental health care use in children. JAMA Pediatr 2019;173:389–91.

12. Cutler GJ, Rodean J, Zima BT, et al. Trends in pediatric emergency department visits for mental health conditions and disposition by presence of a psychiatric unit. Acad Pediatr 2019;19:948–55.

13. Leon SL, Cloutier P, Polihronis C, et al. Child and adolescent mental health repeat visits to the emergency department: a systematic review. Hosp Pediatr 2017;7:177–86.

14. Santiago LI, Tunik MG, Foltin GL, et al. Children requiring psychiatric consultation in the pediatric emergency department: epidemiology, resource utilization, and complications. Pediatr Emerg Care 2006;22(2):85–9. https://doi.org/10.1097/01.pec.0000199568.94758.6e. PMID: 16481922.

15. Gill PJ, Saunders N, Gandhi S, et al. Emergency department as a first contact for mental health problems in children and youth. J Am Acad Child Adolesc Psychiatry 2017;56:475–82.e4.

16. Dell'Osso B, Glick ID, Baldwin DS, et al. Can long-term outcomes be improved by shortening the duration of untreated illness in psychiatric disorders? A conceptual framework. Psychopathology 2013;46:14–21.

17. Steinman KJ, Shoben AB, Dembe AE, et al. How long do adolescents wait for psychiatry appointments? Community Ment Health J 2015;51:782–9.

18. Sheridan DC, Marshall R, Morales AN, et al. Access to outpatient pediatric mental health care after emergency department discharge. Pediatr Emerg Care 2020. https://doi.org/10.1097/PEC.0000000000002057.

19. Lo CB, Bridge JA, Shi J, et al. Children's mental health emergency department visits: 2007-2016. Pediatrics 2020;145:e20191536.

20. Doupnik SK, Esposito J, Lavelle J. Beyond mental health crisis stabilization in emergency departments and acute care hospitals. Pediatrics 2018;141:e20173059.

21. Janiak BD, Atteberry S. Medical clearance of the psychiatric patient in the emergency department. J Emerg Med 2012;43:866–70.

22. Conigliaro A, Benabbas R, Schnitzer E, et al. Protocolized laboratory screening for the medical clearance of psychiatric patients in the emergency department: a systematic review. Acad Emerg Med 2018;25:566–76.

23. Donofrio JJ, Santillanes G, McCammack BD, et al. Clinical utility of screening laboratory tests in pediatric psychiatric patients presenting to the emergency department for medical clearance. Ann Emerg Med

24. Chun TH, Mace SE, Katz ER. American Academy of Pediatrics, Committee on Pediatric Emergency Medicine, American College of Emergency Physicians.

Evaluation and management of children and adolescents with acute mental health or behavioral problems. Part I: Common clinical challenges of patients with mental health and/or behavioral emergencies. Pediatrics 2016;138: e20161570, 2014;63:666-675.e3.

25. Swift RH, Harrigan EP, Cappelleri JC, et al. Validation of the behavioural activity rating scale (BARS): a novel measure of activity in agitated patients. J Psychiatr Res 2002;36(2):87–95.

26. Richmond JS, Berlin JS, Fishkind AB, et al. Verbal de-escalation of the agitated patient: consensus statement of the american association for emergency psychiatry project BETA de-escalation workgroup. West J Emerg Med 2012 Feb;13(1): 17–25.

27. Systematic Review: The Measurement Properties of the Children's Depression Rating Scale-Revised in Adolescents With Major Depressive Disorder.

28. Stallwood E, Monsour A, Rodrigues C, et al. Systematic review: the measurement properties of the children's depression rating scale–revised in adolescents with major depressive disorder. J Am Acad Child Adolesc Psychiatry 2021;60(1): 119–33.

29. Whitfill T, Auerbach M, Scherzer DJ, et al. Emergency care for children in the United States: Epidemiology and trends over time. J Emerg Med 2018;55: 423–34.

Eating Disorders

Diane L. Gorgas, MD

KEYWORDS

- Anorexia • Bulimia • Eating disorders • Purging • Malnutrition

KEY POINTS

- Anorexia nervosa (AN) and bulimia nervosa (BN) are common psychiatric disorders, which can easily be missed in the emergency setting. It is important to recognize the signs and symptoms of the diseases because they have the highest associated mortality of any psychiatric diagnoses.
- Patients with eating disorders use emergency departments for much of their care, and realizing the financial, psychosocial, and physical impacts of correctly managing eating disorders in the ED should be a focus of every emergency provider.
- AN and BN sit in a spectrum of disease and many patients will vacillate in time between the two disorders. The key differences between the diagnoses are caloric restriction and increased caloric expenditure in AN versus caloric purging, sometimes associated with binge eating in BN. Both have a shared component of body dysmorphism and associated psychiatric comorbidities.
- Psychosocial stressors, especially global pandemics leading to increased isolation (COVID 2000-present), impact rates and severity of disease.

INTRODUCTION

Although presenting clinically very differently, eating disorders are unified as a set of psychological disorders in which the patient develops a pathologic relationship with food. The major categories of eating disorders, (1) calorie restrictive disorders (anorexia nervosa [AN]) and (2) binge or binge/purge eating disorders (bulimia nervosa [BN], binge eating disorder [BED], or loss of control [LOC] Eating disorder), are discussed in separate categories here because (1) their prognosis and treatments are very different and (2) within a given episode, the diagnoses are mutually exclusive. Individuals may move between eating disorders and the state of caloric restriction disorder versus those who may binge and purge over time.

Eating disorders of all types are common as comorbid conditions of patients presenting for emergency conditions. In a study screening all ED patients, regardless of presenting symptom, 16% of 1700 patients screened positive for an eating disorder,

Department of Emergency Medicine, Health Sciences Center for Global Health, The Ohio State University, Prior Hall, Floor 7376 West Tenth Avenue, Colubus, OH 43210, USA
E-mail address: Diane.Gorgas@osumc.edu

Emerg Med Clin N Am 42 (2024) 163–179
https://doi.org/10.1016/j.emc.2023.06.024
0733-8627/24/© 2023 Elsevier Inc. All rights reserved.
emed.theclinics.com

with highest correlates noted in female patents and those with concurrent depressive symptoms.[1]

Eating disorders can be challenging to diagnose in the emergency department unless the disease has progressed causing medical complications. Further emphasis is warranted on the topic given a documented lack of focused curricular time spent on eating disorders in emergency medicine (EM) training programs. A study by Trent and colleagues cited 1.9% of residents and faculty in EM completed a rotation focused on eating disorders and 93% of respondents were unfamiliar with the American Psychiatric Association's Practice Guideline for the Treatment of Patients with Eating Disorders. In a limited survey sample, most of the respondents desired more education on eating disorders, specifically focused on assessment, complications, and criteria for hospitalization.[2] This is further emphasized by Redekopp's work showing that.

Eating disorder patients are discharged from the emergency department without follow-up being arranged for their eating disorder 68.7% of the time.[3] The lack of appropriate referral for treatment was posited to be multifactorial including (1) lack of recognition of the disorder itself and (2) lack of systems knowledge in resources and appropriate referral patterns. The study highlighted a need for better early detection but also a more interdisciplinary and structural awareness of resources available to patients with eating disorders.

This article strives to improve emergency physicians' ability to diagnose subtle cases of eating disorders, discusses medically apparent ED complications, and touches on treatment.

The financial impact of eating disorders on the medical system is significant. Financial impact of eating disorders in a British study are estimated as $2993 to 67,000 USD annually, but these numbers rarely included specific treatment aimed at the core disorder and instead focus on management of complications. Rarely were the majority of these expenditures focused on long-term efforts for recovery, but rather a large proportion of this was managing medical complications of eating disorders.[4] Beyond the financial impacts, Health related Quality of Life for patients diagnosed with eating disorders is seriously impacted. Estimates are that annually over 3.3 million healthy life years worldwide are lost because of eating disorders. In contrast to other mental health disorders, there has been an increased years lived with disability with eating disorders. Despite treatment advances, mortality rates of AN and BN remain very high. Those who have received inpatient treatment for AN still have a more than five times increased mortality risk.

ANOREXIA NERVOSA
Definition

AN is a complex psychological disease with a unified manifestation of severe caloric restriction relative to requirements and/or efforts at caloric wasting/elimination leading to a low body mass index. This is defined as restrictive versus binge/purge AN with combinations of both in a single patient (binge mechanisms will be discussed under Bulimia section) Previous Diagnostic and Statistical Manual of Mental Health (DSM) versions divided avoidant/restrictive food intake disorder, rumination disorder, and pica as purely pediatric conditions, but the latest edition DSM-5[5] rolls these diagnoses into either AN, BN, or BED. Common in the symptom complex associated with AN is body dysmorphism, a fixed delusional derangement of the ability to view self-evaluation of body weight objectively. Body dysmorphism is associated with a fear of gaining weight and an associated disturbance in body image.

The condition is further characterized by differentiating those who achieve their weight loss predominantly through restricting intake or by excessive exercise from those who engage in recurrent binge eating and/or subsequent purging, self-induced vomiting, and usage of enemas, laxatives, or diuretics (binge eating/purging type). There is frequently a denial of the consequences of very low BMI and the cause and effect between caloric restriction and physical symptoms. The goal of continued weight loss is the perpetual and sole focus for these patients, and logic in plotting out their weight trajectory or explaining harmful sequelae of caloric restriction or excessive physical activity is ineffective. At a point in the illness, the malnutrition affects cognitive processing and the disparities of objective health and desired body morphology and goals widen.

Although currently classified as a functional disorder within psychiatry, there is a familial heritability in AN and a chromosomal abnormality which has been mapped (rs4622308). Processing abnormalities have been noted on functional MRIs in AN patients.

Incidence/Prevalence

The prevalence of AN in the United States is up to 4%, with a strong gender propensity where women and girls are affected much more than men and boys. The lifetime prevalence for AN, BN, and BED diagnoses are higher among sexual and gender minority adolescents and adults compared with cisgender heterosexuals in the United States. Lifetime prevalence of eating disorders is 10.5% for transgender men and 8.1% for transgender women in the United States.[6] Men account for 10% of all AN cases, but the disorder is likely underdiagnosed in men and boys. Male goals in the disease tend to focus more on adding muscle mass and decreasing adiposity, most associated with antecedent obesity, athletic performance concerns, and being the victim of bullying. Highly suggestive evidence supported the association between childhood sexual abuse and BN and between appearance-related teasing victimization and any eating disorder.[7] The onset is typically in adolescence, but adult cases can occur.

The COVID pandemic seems to have impacted the incidence of AN and risk of complications from the disorder.[8] A cross-sectional study found a higher number of new diagnoses of and hospitalizations for AN or atypical AN in children and adolescents during the first wave of the COVID-19 pandemic in Canada.

Given the incidence and prevalence of the disease and the myriad of medical complications associated with eating disorders, it is important that emergency physicians understand the presenting concerns, can identify the physical findings, and recognize complications associated with eating disorders.[9]

Presentation

History

The presentation of a patient in the early stages of AN is generally vague. Early to midstage presenting symptoms include fatigue, lightheadedness or syncope, insomnia, weakness, pallor, or confusion. Nausea and vomiting are common yet a challenging presenting symptoms because attributing these symptoms to the cause of low body mass index (BMI) versus a consequence of the AN itself is frequently difficult to untangle.

The goal of survey assessment is to understand the patient's goals and behaviors focused on those listed in **Boxes 1** and **2**.[10]

This survey has been distilled into a brief evaluation tool (the SCOFF index) which can be used in EM and outpatient settings.

Extracurricular hobbies and sports which are associated but not causative of AN include gymnastics, ballet, dance, wrestling, swimming, and cross-country running.[11]

Box 1
Behavioral and psychological risks for AN

Eating and dieting behavior

Desire for weight loss

Body morphology self-assessment

History of caloric counting, food portion control

Use of laxatives or purge mechanisms

History of food avoidance

Goal-oriented exercise

Physical Examination Findings

The most common sign of AN is a low BMI (< 18.5). If AN is suspected, an accurate height and weight should be obtained for primary diagnosis but also for tracking of disease progression. Self-reporting of these vital statistics is unreliable and not warranted and every effort should be taken to directly measure height and weight.

Vital sign abnormalities are the rule rather than the exception when the BMI drops below 16 and are characterized by hypotension, hypothermia, and most commonly bradycardia, although tachycardia may be present. AN patients can develop impaired thermoregulation resulting in acrocyanosis (**Fig. 1**). Brittle fragile nails can also be noted.

Other morphologic manifestations include the presence of lanugo a fine, long hair on the arms and face (**Fig. 2**).

The oral examination may demonstrate signs of malnutrition including stomatitis or cheilitis or alternatively may show consequences of purging behavior (see section on Bulimia).

Associations with mental health disorders are common in patients with AN. Preexisting mental health disorders, specifically anxiety and obsessive-compulsive disorder, are common. A thorough skin examination, noting evidence of self-injurious behavior and episodic cutting should be documented. This should include upper and lower extremities (**Fig. 3**).

Comorbid Pathologies and Emergency Complications

It is essential for emergency medicine physicians to know that AN can be a life-threatening condition, even in its early stages.

Box 2
The SCOFF index: questions for patients

The SCOFF questions[a]

Do you make yourself Sick because you feel uncomfortably full?

Do you worry you have lost Control over how much you eat?

Have you recently lost more than (Over) *15 lbs* in a 3 month period?

Do you believe yourself to be Fat when others say you are too thin?

Would you say that Food dominates your life?

[a]One point for every "yes"; a score of $\not\geq 2$ indicates a likely case of anorexia nervosa or bulimia

---

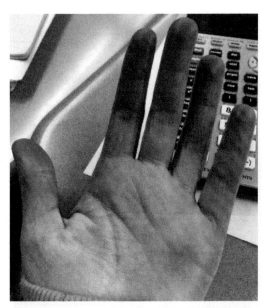

Fig. 1. Demonstration of acrocyanosis (Gorgas).

Patients manifesting even the early stages of AN can have significant psychiatric risks, including *five to six times* the risk of suicide compared with non-AN age compared cohorts. As already outlined, self-injurious behavior or self-cutting have been documented as risk characteristics for suicide completion.

The physical complications of later stage AN, generally associated with malnutrition, are outlined below. These include:

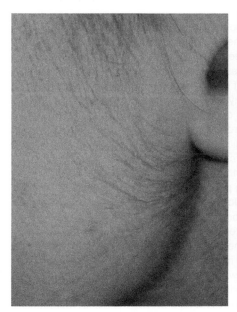
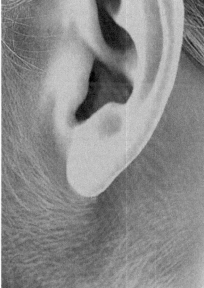

Fig. 2. Lanugo: a fine long hair growth common on the face and arms (credit Gorgas).

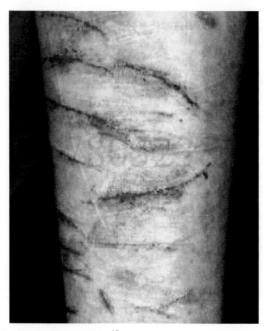

Fig. 3. Evidence of self-injurious cutting.[12]

Cardiac: The severity of hypotension, orthostasis, and bradycardia can be mapped directly to the severity of malnutrition and low BMI. These complications result from decreased cardiac muscle mass accompanied by increased vagal tone, thus worsening risks for syncope. Chest radiography may reveal a small cardiac silhouette.

Cardiac contractility can be noted on point-of-care ultrasound or through echocardiography. Other cardiac abnormalities seen in AN as compared with healthy controls were reduced left ventricular mass, reduced cardiac output, and increased incidence of pericardial effusions.[13,14] Myocardial wasting can lead to mitral valve prolapse. Cardiac dysfunction is augmented if syrup of ipecac is used in purging behaviors, since emetine, its main ingredient is a direct myocardial toxin. The production of syrup of ipecac ceased in 2010, so toxicity is less commonly noted now.

QT prolongation can be noted on electrocardiogram (ECG) and is a sign of cardiac irritability and increased risk of dysrhythmias. A prolonged QTC is almost always seen with bradycardia less than 60 beats per minute (BPM).[15]

Pulmonary complications are more common in patients who undertake purging and forced emesis, but general malnutrition in patients with AN can cause weakened diaphragmatic musculature and weakened glottic and pharyngeal muscles. These conditions lead to the increased risk of pulmonary infection given a lack of capacity for productive coughing and aspiration of even saliva and water.[16]

Endocrine: Hypothalamic-mediated amenorrhea is very common and is one of the commonly used diagnostic criteria for AN in girls and women. Other endocrine conditions seen are "euthyroid sick syndrome" where the thyroid stimulating hormone (TSH) level is normal or slightly low, T3 is low, and T4 may either be low or normal. High levels of cortisol and low levels of insulin-like growth factor increase the risk of malnutrition-associated osteoporosis.[17]

A well-documented paradoxic hyperlipidemia with increased total cholesterol levels exceeding 300 to 400 is seen, which generally corrects with weight gain.

Electrolyte and Renal: The most common constellation of electrolyte abnormalities in calorific restrictive AN (not purging) is starvation ketosis, hypoglycemia, and hypophosphatemia. Hypovolemia associated with oral restrictive behaviors can lead to acute kidney injury.

Gastrointestinal (GI) catastrophes are uncommon in AN, but the emergency provider should be aware of some with life-threatening potential.

There are cases of gastric dilation and gastric necrosis with rupture.[18] Gastric distension due to chronic gastric motility is thought to originate from initial binge and purge behaviors with secondary exacerbation by general malnutrition. In end-stage cases, gastric distension not related to food intake has been well documented.[19] Gastric distension can become so severe as to cause acute renal failure[20] or limb ischemia[21] by direct compression of surrounding structures. Rare cases of death from aortic compression have been reported (**Fig. 4**).[22]

Hung-Hao Fan published a case report of massive ascites (even in the setting of normal albumin and no proteinuria)[23] More typically, gastric dysmotility and intolerance of refeeding are common complications seen during the treatment phase of AN.

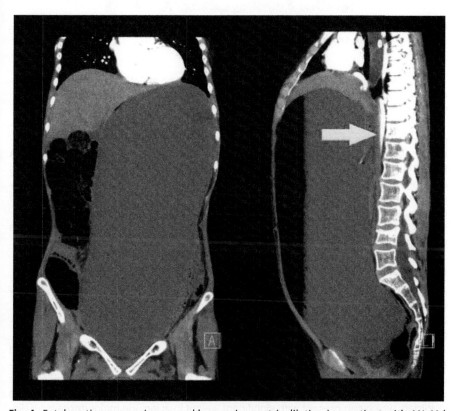

Fig. 4. Fatal aortic compression caused by massive gastric dilation in a patient with AN. *Yellow arrow* demonstrates aortic compression with termination of contrast in the lower thoracic region. (Enzmann F, Guggenbichler S. Fatal Aortic Occlusion Due to Compression From Self Induced Acute Gastric Dilatation. Eur J Vasc Endovasc Surg. 2019 Aug;58(2):281. https://doi.org/10.1016/j.ejvs.2019.02.025. Epub 2019 Jun 17. PMID: 31221538.)

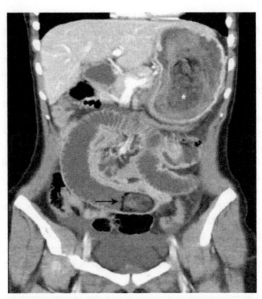

Fig. 5. Trichobezoar in a patient with AN causing an obstruction.[24] *Black arrow* demonstrates trichobezoar causing obstruction.

Pica or the ingestion of noncaloric substances can be an intentional behavior in patients with AN as a method to staunch hunger. Pica can cause gastric outlet obstruction and small bowel obstructions in the development of bezoars (**Fig. 5**).

Attempts at weight gain by refeeding can also be significantly complicated by superior mesenteric artery (SMA) syndrome. In AN, this is caused by loss of intra-abdominal adiposity which can in turn result in an acute angle take off of the SMA from the aorta. SMA syndrome makes refeeding exceedingly difficult, as attempts at using an enteric route for nutrition can lead to severe abdominal pain (caused by demand mesenteric ischemia), nausea, and vomiting. In severe cases, parenteral nutrition needs to be given until a critical amount of intra-abdominal adiposity develops to lessen the angle of takeoff of the SMA from the aorta, improving symptoms and allowing for initiation of enteral feeds.[25]

Differential Diagnosis

AN and BN are the new "great masqueraders."[26] Care should be taken to consider other wasting disorders when making the diagnosis of AN including HIV, tuberculosis, adrenal insufficiency (primary), hyperthyroidism, diabetes, celiac disease, inflammatory bowel disease, and primary SMA syndrome.

A laboratory workup to help rule out primary causes of severe weight loss should include testing for mononucleosis, pregnancy (given potentially undiagnosed hyperemesis gravidarum), substance use disorder (SUD), inflammatory bowel disease or possible irritable bowel disorder with food avoidance, and SMA syndrome. Psychiatric disorders which can present with significant weight loss include major depressive disorder, bipolar disorder, and schizophrenia.

Diagnostic studies in cases of suspected AN with low BMI include an ECG to evaluate heart rate and QT intervals, and a comprehensive metabolic panel to rule out hypo- and hyperglycemia, abnormal renal function, and abnormal results of magnesium, calcium, and phosphate levels (all common derangements in AN). A urinalysis should be collected and tested for proteinuria as well as a complete blood count to rule out anemia and pancytopenia associated with malnutrition. Serum albumin, liver function tests, and a lipase level should be obtained as each of these can be abnormal in starvation states. Thyroid function testing is important to help rule out severe hyperthyroidism as a cause of malnutrition (even though tachycardia is more common with thyroid disease and bradycardia with AN, this is not a hard and fast rule) but also to screen for euthyroid sick syndrome. Imaging is only helpful to rule out other causes of the wasting disorder or in consideration of severe complications on presentation (bowel obstruction/ileus, gastric dilation, heart failure, and so forth) or when considering central causes of hyperemesis and malnutrition (increased intracranial pressure secondary to central nervous system [CNS] neoplastic disease).

Disposition

Initial considerations for treatment of AN patients include selecting a proper disposition for the acute on chronically ill patient. The Society of Adolescent Medicine has set criteria for in-patient admission which are listed in **Box 3**.

Patients who are determined to not meet inpatient criteria may be discharged to home if care coordination and follow-up is assured from the emergency department. Every effort should be made to establish care if patients do not have a preexisting relationship with a primary care physician and psychiatrist/psychologist. A multidisciplinary approach including follow-up with a counselor, nutritionist, and medical specialists is also needed for successful long-term outcomes.

Treatment

The mainstay of long-term AN treatment is focused on cognitive/behavioral therapy (CBT). An example of this is the MANTRA or Maudsley AN Treatment for Adults protocol,[28] which consists of seven core modules conducted over 20 to 40 sessions. This treatment plan aims to address the cognitive, emotional, relational, and biological factors which tend to anchor wasting behaviors by working out what prevents progression in treating anorexia. The program is designed to allow the patient to find more adaptive and alternate ways of coping.

Box 3
Society of Adolescent Medicine criteria for in-patient admission for AN[27]

Body weight less than 75% of ideal for age, sex, height

Body fat less than 10% of body weight

Vital Sign Abnormalities:
  Awake pulse less than 50 BPM or sleeping $P < 45$ BPM
  Temp less than 96 F
  Systolic blood pressure less than 90 mm Hg

General: Dehydration

Cardiac: arrhythmias including prolonged QT intervals

Orthostasis and syncope

Failure of outpatient treatment (ongoing weight loss or failure of weight gain despite treatment)

Psychiatric: suicidality, hallucinations

Environmental Concerns: lack of family support, structure, and so forth

Unfortunately, there is no pharmacologic "silver bullet" which has been proven successful in treating AN. Associated depression and anxiety should be treated with standard regimens.

Structured refeeding programs are necessary therapy in moderate to severe disease. In conjunction with CBT programs, this may initially consist of placement of feeding tubes or even bridging parenteral nutrition to provide enough nutrition to slowly reengage peristalsis and gut motility and manage symptoms of SMA syndrome. The goal of a refeeding program is slow, gradual progress with ideal weight gain goals of 0.5 to 1.0 lb per week. Refeeding is a vulnerable physiologic time for complications and electrolytes should be closely monitored. The literature has case reports of hyperglycemia and subsequent torsades des pointes as a complication of refeeding.[29]

Prognosis

Overall, long-term prognosis of the disease is good, but remission rates of 70% to 80% in adulthood are noted if onset was in adolescence.[30] There is significant variability in the progress and recovery from the disorder. The natural course of the disorder sees some individuals recovering after a single episode, yet others carrying the diagnosis and requiring treatment for life. Treatment is essential because AN has a mortality of 5.1/1000, the highest among all psychiatric conditions.[31] Some studies cite the risk of suicide as high as x12 compared with age and socioeconomically matched cohorts, yielding an absolute rate for those carrying the diagnosis as 4% to 11% over a lifetime.

Most of the cardiac sequelae of AN are reversible after a successful refeeding program with the exception of syrup of ipecac associated direct myocardial toxicity and rare cases of myocardial fibrosis. The resolution of bradycardia and normalization of QT intervals has been a reliable marker for success of refeeding programs, often preceding increased BMI.

BULIMIA AND BINGE-EATING DISORDER

Bulimia or BN differs from AN in that patients (1) may have a low, normal, or increased BMI and (2) their relationship with food is associated with bringing and purging of calories, either through emesis or increased motility and laxative/colon cleansing.

BED is similar to BN in that bingeing is a key component, but differs in that there are no compensatory behaviors to prevent weight gain. There are similarities in distress over the eating patterns and often a disconnect between binge eating and other health conditions and physical symptoms. There is an overwhelming experience of LOC leading to its alternative label of LOC eating disorder. This manifests in eating more rapidly or in greater amounts than intended or eating when not hungry. The 12-month prevalence in females is 1.6%, with a much lower female-to-male ratio than BN. Little is known about the course of the disorder, given its recent categorization, but its prognosis is markedly better than for other eating disorders, both in terms of its natural course and response to treatment. Transition to other eating disorder conditions is thought to be rare.

Incidence/Prevalence

Men and boys account for 25% of patients with BN.[1] Screening positive for BN is most commonly associated with a BMI over 30 in the ED, illustrating a key difference from AN. This section will not only consider BN but also BED (aka LOC eating disorder). The prevalence of BN in a study in the pediatric population was 22%, whereas BED was seen in as high as 31% of cases.[32]

The risk factors for development of BN and BED are similar to those of AN, but there is an even stronger association with childhood sexual abuse.[7]

There is an association of general SUDs, most notably with tobacco use disorder and habitual cocaine users.[33,34]

Spectrum

It is important to recall that although the discussion of these disorders is separated in this article, BN, AN, and BED can represent a continuum along the spectrum of eating disorders and some patients can move between the diagnoses over time. Up to 50% of anorexic patients develop bulimia.

Presentation

History can be confounding in diagnosing BN and BED because patients are rarely forthcoming with respect to their eating and purging patterns, but GI symptoms, generalized weakness, and oral complaints are the most common presenting concerns. As with AN, denial of symptoms and behaviors is a common feature and patients as a rule frequently do not see an association between purging behaviors and their presenting concerns.

Physical Examination

General: Patients presenting with BN are generally well-groomed with good hygiene. Their BMI may be low, normal, or high.

Ear, Nose, Throat: Key to the diagnosis of BN is a thorough oral examination. Common features associated with long-standing self-induced purging include dental erosions or early dental enamel discoloration and dysplasia. (**Figs. 6 and 7**) This is a direct effect of exposure to gastric acid.

Bruises and lacerations of posterior pharynx can be seen as a result of self-induced gagging with fingers or any other foreign body. These are can be noted on the posterior soft palate or on the contralateral side of hand dominance around the tonsillar pillars and uvula. Pyorrhea and other gum disorders can also be noted. Parotitis and diffuse salivary gland hyperplasia can be observed and will be tender on palpation[35] (**Fig. 8**).

Extremities

The practice of repeated self-induced emesis using the fingers and hand can caused scars or callus formation over the dorsal surface of the hands (Russell's sign) (**Fig. 9**). The extremity examination may also demonstrate generalized or localized edema of lower extremities.

Pulmonary

Much like in AN, aspiration pneumonia can be seen but is usually associated with purging behavior and not intrinsic diaphragmatic and glottic weakness. Shortness of breath may also occur associated with severe hypokalemia and smooth muscle paralysis. Repeated emesis and laryngoesophageal reflux can cause chronic hoarseness and dysphagia. Less common physical findings may point to the diagnosis of pneumomediastinum from forced emesis or membranous tracheal stenosis.[29] There are also rare reports of pneumothorax.

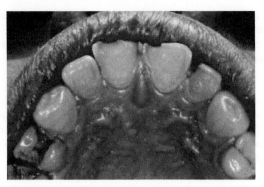

Fig. 6. Demonstration of the loss of enamel in the lingual surface of the upper incisors after purging and enamel exposure to gastric acid.[36]

GASTROINTESTINAL

Gastrointestinal findings include ileus with abdominal distension. Mallory Weiss tears are relatively commonly seen, but Boerhaave syndrome rarely occurs. Purging via chronic stimulant/laxative abuse can lead to ileus, rectal prolapse, melanosis coli, and cathartic colon syndrome.

Acute gastric dilatation may be noted and attributable to electrolyte abnormalities but may also be associated with binge eating.[39]

Additional Physical Findings

Other physical findings in patients with purging behaviors are usually associated with the moderate to severe metabolic and electrolyte derangements. Hypotension and a weak pulse may be noted because of hypovolemia. Dysrhythmias and decreased cardiac output, along with poor-quality heart sounds and shortness of breath, may all be associated with severe hypokalemia.

Neurologic findings associated with severe hypokalemia and hypocalcemia include muscle cramping (Trousseau's sign), diminished reflexes, muscle weakness, and paralysis.

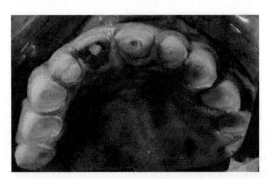

Fig. 7. Severe dental erosion as a result of prolonged history of purging.[37]

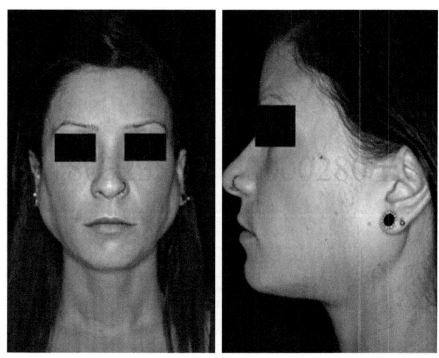

Fig. 8. Parotitis in a patient with BN and purging.[36]

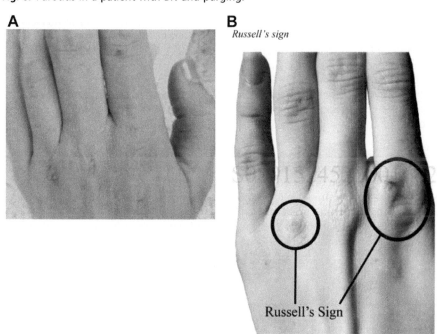

Fig. 9. Scars and callouses over the dorsum of the L hand in a patient with bulimia and self-induced emesis. (Credit: *A*: Gorgas; *B*: Chew).[38] (Russell's Sign on the knuckles of the index and ring fingers. By Kyukyusha. Retrieved from: https://commons.wikimedia.org/w/index.php?curid=5053797.)

> **Box 4**
> **Laboratory findings in bulimia**
>
> Metabolic alkalosis (hypochloremia, elevated serum bicarbonate)
>
> Hypokalemia (secondary to metabolic alkalosis)
>
> Hypovolemia with secondary hyperaldosteronism (also contributes to hypokalemia), pseudo-Bartter's syndrome
>
> Bulimia with vomiting and purging (laxatives or diuretics)
>
> All the above findings, plus:
>
> Decreased body potassium and body sodium secondary to diarrhea and renal losses
>
> Metabolic acidosis with spuriously normal serum potassium
>
> Hypokalemic nephropathy (urine concentrating deficit)
>
> Hypokalemic myopathy (including cardiomyopathy)
>
> Hypocalcemia or hypercalcemia, hypomagnesemia, hypophosphatemia

Laboratory Findings

Laboratory findings in bulimia are associated with severe gastric fluid and electrolyte loss with purging, including self-induced emesis and laxative abuse. These are outlined in **Box 4**.

Patients with BN also have an increased incidence of hyperlipidemia, diabetes mellitus (DM) 1 and DM 2, and hyperaldosteronism.

Treatment

Unlike AN, pharmacologic treatment for primary bulimia (as opposed to associated psychiatric comorbidities of anxiety and depression in AN) is effective. Specifically, fluoxetine for BN and lisdexamfetamine for BED are relatively safe and well tolerated. Pharmacologic adjuncts to CBT have the potential to improve long-term compliance and patient commitment to treatment for eating disorders[40] Other pharmacologic treatments include topiramate, antidepressants, and anti-obesity drugs. Each of these off-label treatments has been explored for the treatment of BN and BED with variable success.

Prognosis

There are noted predictors for the rate of rapid relapse of BN and BED including higher frequencies of bingeing and vomiting before treatment and engaging in less body avoidance before treatment. Weight and shape concerns (including body checking) were not associated with rapid relapse.

The 68.2% of participants with BN recover at 9-year follow-up, and this rate holds for studies looking out to 20- and 22-year post-diagnosis.[41]

CLINICS CARE POINTS

- The SCOFF Survey is a brief, five-question tool which can be used even in busy clinical settings to help screen for AN as a primary rather than secondary cause of significant weight loss/low BMI.
- Physical findings of AN, including a low BMI defined as less than 18, include general findings of malnutrition (acrocyanosis, lanugo, cheilitis, and low cardiac mass and contractility).

- Cardiac complications in AN include syncope with marked bradycardia and QT prolongation with an increased risk of dysrhythmias. Electrolyte disturbances, particularly during the refeeding phase, can exacerbate these complications.

- Emergency physicians may have a significantly more challenging time in diagnosing BN, because patients may present with either low, normal, or increased BMI. Careful examination for signs of purging, either orally through induced emesis or fecally through excessive use of laxatives and promotility agents, is important. Careful examination for and documentation of dental erosions, posterior oropharyngeal bruising, Russel's sign, and salivary and parotid gland inflammation are clues to the purging behavior.

- Treatment for AN should include cognitive behavioral therapy with concomitant efforts to treat any psychiatric comorbidities (often anxiety, obsessive-compulsive disorder, and depression), whereas BN and BED have been successfully treated with fluoxetine and lisdexamfetamine, respectively.

DISCLOSURE

The author has nothing to disclose.

REFERENCES

1. Ernest S, Kuntz HM. Emergency department management of eating disorder complications in pediatric patients. Pediatr Emerg Med Pract 2020;17(2):1–16. https://www.ncbi.nlm.nih.gov/pubmed/31978295.
2. Ma C, Gonzales-Pacheco D, Cerami J, et al. Emergency medicine physicians' knowledge and perceptions of training, education, and resources in eating disorders. Journal of eating disorders 2021;9(1):4. https://www.ncbi.nlm.nih.gov/pubmed/33407918.
3. Redekopp C, Dimitropoulos G, Patten S, et al. Considering a risk profile based on emergency department utilization in young people with eating disorders: Implications for early detection. Int J Eat Disord 2022;55(9):1219–28. https://onlinelibrary.wiley.com/doi/abs/10.1002/eat.23588.
4. Ágh T, Kovács G, Supina D, et al. A systematic review of the health-related quality of life and economic burdens of anorexia nervosa, bulimia nervosa, and binge eating disorder. Eat Weight Disord 2016;21(3):353–64. https://link.springer.com/article/10.1007/s40519-016-0264-x.
5. American Psychiatric Association. Diagnostic and statistical manual of mental disorders. 5th edition. Washington, DC: American Psychiatric Association Publishing; 2022. text revision ed.
6. Nagata J, Ganson K, Austin S. Emerging trends in eating disorders among sexual and gender minorities. Curr Opin Psychiatr 2020;33(6):562–7. https://www.ncbi.nlm.nih.gov/pubmed/32858597.
7. Solmi M, Radua J, Stubbs B, et al. Risk factors for eating disorders: An umbrella review of published meta-analyses. Rev Bras Psiquiatr 2021;43(3):314–23. https://search.proquest.com/docview/2447542676.
8. Agostino H, Burstein B, Moubayed D, et al. Trends in the incidence of new-onset anorexia nervosa and atypical anorexia nervosa among youth during the COVID-19 pandemic in canada. JAMA Netw Open 2021;4(12):e2137395.
9. Mascolo M, Trent S, Colwell C, et al. What the emergency department needs to know when caring for your patients with eating disorders. Int J Eat Disord 2012;45(8):977–81. https://api.istex.fr/ark:/67375/WNG-JJFJ595Z-5/fulltext.pdf.

10. Kutz AM, Marsh AG, Gunderson CG, et al. Eating disorder screening: A systematic review and meta-analysis of diagnostic test characteristics of the SCOFF. J Gen Intern Med 2020;35(3):885–93. https://link.springer.com/article/10.1007/s11606-019-05478-6.

11. Sudi K, Öttl K, Payerl D, et al. Anorexia athletica. Nutrition 2004;20(7):657–61.

12. Innes JA, Dover AR, Fairhurst K. Macleod's clinical examination. Philadelphia: Elsevier; 2018. https://ebookcentral.proquest.com/lib/[SITE_ID]/detail.action?docID=5434816.

13. Smythe J, Colebourn C, Prisco L, et al. Cardiac abnormalities identified with echocardiography in anorexia nervosa: Systematic review and meta-analysis. Br J Psychiatr 2021;219(3):477–86.

14. Spina G, Roversi M, Marchili MR, et al. Psychiatric comorbidities and dehydration are more common in children admitted to the emergency department for eating disorders in the COVID-19 era. Eat Weight Disord 2022;27(7):2473–80. https://link.springer.com/article/10.1007/s40519-022-01386-7.

15. Ajam M, Abu-Heija AA, Shokr M, et al. Sinus bradycardia and QT interval prolongation in west nile virus encephalitis: A case report. Cureus 2019;11(1):e3821. https://www.ncbi.nlm.nih.gov/pubmed/30868034.

16. Solomon N, Sailer A, Dixe de Oliveira Santo I, et al. Sequelae of eating disorders at imaging. Radiographics 2022;42(5):1377–97. https://search.proquest.com/docview/2699704956.

17. Bowden DJ, Kilburn-Toppin F, Scoffings DJ. Radiology of eating disorders: A pictorial review. Radiographics 2013;33(4):1171–93. https://www.ncbi.nlm.nih.gov/pubmed/23842978.

18. Swed S, Ezzdean W, Sawaf B. Chronic gastric dilatation with gastric fundus perforation in anorexia nervosa patient. International journal of surgery case reports 2022;90:106645.

19. Panyko A, Vician M, Dubovský M. Massive acute gastric dilatation in a patient with anorexia nervosa. J Gastrointest Surg 2021;25(3):856–8. https://link.springer.com/article/10.1007/s11605-020-04715-2.

20. Dumouchel J, Lvovschi V, et al. Obstructive acute renal failure by severe gastric distension after binge. Am J Emerg Med 2017;35(8):1210, e5-1210.e7. https://www.clinicalkey.es/playcontent/1-s2.0-S0735675717302140.

21. Van Eetvelde E, Verfaillie L, et al. Acute gastric dilatation causing acute limb ischemia in an Anorexia Nervosa patient. J Emerg Med 2014;46(5):e141–3. https://www.clinicalkey.es/playcontent/1-s2.0-S0736467913014194.

22. Enzmann F, Guggenbichler S. Fatal aortic occlusion due to compression from self-induced acute gastric dilatation. Eur J Vasc Endovasc Surg 2019;58(2):281.

23. Fan H, Lin I, Chen J, et al. Anorexia nervosa manifesting as massive ascites, hypercholesterolemia, and sequential binge eating in an 11-year-old girl: A case report. Medicine (Baltim) 2020;99(35):e21739. https://www.ncbi.nlm.nih.gov/pubmed/32871893.

24. Coley B. Caffey's pediatric diagnostic imaging. 12th edition. Elsevier Health Sciences; 2013. 2 vol set. http://www.r2library.com/resource/title/9780323081764.

25. Watters A, Gibson D, Dee E, et al. Superior mesenteric artery syndrome in severe anorexia nervosa: A case series. Clinical Case Reports 2020;8(1):185–9. https://onlinelibrary.wiley.com/doi/abs/10.1002/ccr3.2577.

26. Trent SA, Moreira ME, et al. ED management of patients with eating disorders. Am J Emerg Med 2013;31(5):859–65. https://www.clinicalkey.es/playcontent/1-s2.0-S073567571300140X.

27. Tintinalli JE, Ma OJ, Yealy DM, et al. Tintinalli's emergency medicine. 9th edition. New York, N.Y: McGraw-Hill Education LLC; 2020. https://accessmedicine. mhmedical.com/book.aspx?bookid=2353.

28. Wittek T, Truttmann S, Zeiler M, et al. The Maudsley model of anorexia nervosa treatment for adolescents and young adults (MANTRa): A study protocol for a multi-center cohort study. Journal of eating disorders 2021;9(1):33. https://www. ncbi.nlm.nih.gov/pubmed/33685522.

29. Nakashima T, Kubota T, et al. Hyperglycemia and subsequent torsades de pointes with marked QT prolongation during refeeding. Nutrition 2016;33: 145–8. https://www.clinicalkey.es/playcontent/1-s2.0-S0899900716300855.

30. Jagielska G, Kacperska I. Outcome, comorbidity and prognosis in anorexia nervosa. Psychiatr Pol 2017;51(2):205–18. https://www.ncbi.nlm.nih.gov/pubmed/28581532.

31. Pompili M, Mancinelli I, Girardi P, et al. Suicide in anorexia nervosa: A meta-analysis. Int J Eat Disord 2004;36(1):99–103. https://agris.fao.org/agris-search/search.do? recordID=US201300937019.

32. He J, Cai Z, Fan X. Prevalence of binge and loss of control eating among children and adolescents with overweight and obesity: An exploratory meta-analysis. Int J Eat Disord 2017;50(2):91–103. https://onlinelibrary.wiley.com/doi/abs/10.1002/ eat.22661.

33. Munn-Chernoff MA, Johnson EC, Chou Y, et al. Shared genetic risk between eating disorder- and substance-use-related phenotypes: evidence from genome-wide association studies. 2020. http://hdl.handle.net/11250/3037615.

34. Walfish S, Stenmark DE, Sarco D, et al. Incidence of bulimia in substance misusing women in residential treatment. Int J Addict 1992;27(4):425–33. https://www. tandfonline.com/doi/abs/10.3109/10826089209068751.

35. Colella G, Lo Giudice G, De Luca R, et al. Interventional sialendoscopy in parotidomegaly related to eating disorders. Journal of eating disorders 2021;9(1):25. https://www.ncbi.nlm.nih.gov/pubmed/33597023.

36. Little J, Miller C, Rhodus N. Little and falace's dental management of the medically compromised patient. 9th edition. Elsevier Health Sciences; 2018. http:// www.r2library.com/resource/title/9780323443555.

37. Eakle WS, Bastin KG. Dental materials: clinical applications for dental assistants and dental hygienists. Saunders; 2019. https://www.vlebooks.com/vleweb/ product/openreader?id=none&isbn=9780323596596.

38. Chew KK, Temples HS. Adolescent eating disorders: Early identification and management in primary care. J Pediatr Health Care 2022;36(6):618–27. https:// doi.org/10.1016/j.pedhc.2022.06.004.

39. Dincel O, Goksu M. Acute gastric dilatation due to binge eating may be fatal. Northern Clinics of Istanbul 2017;4(2):199–202. https://www.ncbi.nlm.nih.gov/ pubmed/28971182.

40. Bello NT, Yeomans BL. Safety of pharmacotherapy options for bulimia nervosa and binge eating disorder. Expet Opin Drug Saf 2018;17(1):17–23. https://www. tandfonline.com/doi/abs/10.1080/14740338.2018.1395854.

41. Eddy KT, Tabri N, Thomas JJ, et al. Recovery from anorexia nervosa and bulimia nervosa at 22-year follow-up. J Clin Psychiatr 2017;78(2):184–9. https://www. ncbi.nlm.nih.gov/pubmed/28002660.

Difficult Patients
Malingerers, Feigners, Chronic Complainers, and Real Imposters

Artun K. Kadaster, BS[a,1], Markayle R. Schears, MPH[b,*], Raquel M. Schears, MD, MPH, MBA[c]

KEYWORDS

- Malinger • Deception • Exaggerate • ED presentation • Incentive • Identity theft
- Somatic symptom disorder

KEY POINTS

- Difficult patients are often those who present with a mix of psychiatric and physical issues, and may be categorized as malingerers, true feigners, chronic complainers, and/or real imposters.
- The true incidence of malingering in the emergency department (ED) is unknown because it is difficult to ascertain whether patients are fabricating or exaggerating symptoms.
- Malingering is considered a diagnosis of exclusion that involves the intentional simulation or significant exaggeration of symptoms.
- ED management includes remaining neutral, empathetic and avoiding labeling (NEAL) to optimize outcomes for shared medical decision-making.

INTRODUCTION

Malingering is one of the few medical diagnoses often not documented in the medical record, due to the controversy and consequences the labeling may cause patients. Doctors are trained to detect illness and injury patterns and to treat the diseases. Thus, the simulated presentation of an illness or injury is disruptive to the doctor–patient relationship. Once suspected, it has the potential to convert the relationship from one of benevolence to one of antagonism. Mistakenly, some may believe exposing the deception is productive. Often this tactic does not dissuade the malingerer. Currently, a critical knowledge gap exists in establishing an accurate base rate for malingering which is considered to be a necessary first step to developing

[a] Department of Anesthesia, Mayo Clinic –Rochester; [b] University of Wisconsin School of Medicine and Public Health, 750 Highland Avenue, Madison, WI 53705, USA; [c] University of Central Florida, 400 Central Florida Boulevard, Orlando, FL 32816, USA
[1] Present address: 325 9th Street Northwest, Byron, MN 55920.
* Corresponding author.
E-mail address: mschears@wisc.edu

Emerg Med Clin N Am 42 (2024) 181–195
https://doi.org/10.1016/j.emc.2023.06.018
0733-8627/24/© 2023 Elsevier Inc. All rights reserved.
emed.theclinics.com

management strategies. Despite this considerable limitation, the published literature does share plenty of advice on how to unmask malingering. Foremost, the notion to seek clarity over confrontation with patients should guide the physician's approach and may help to mitigate any potential negative reaction.

Malingering is defined as the intentional production of false or grossly exaggerated physical or psychological symptoms, motivated by external incentives such as avoiding work duties or attendance responsibilities, or legal consequences, or obtaining goods and services, such as accommodations in the hospital or financial compensation including disability benefits, or procurement of controlled substances.[1] The Diagnostic and Statistical Manual of Mental Disorders, Fifth Edition (DSM-5) and Eleventh Edition of International Classification of Diseases (ICD-11) have similar definitions of malingering.[1–3] The latest DSM-5-TR carries along the "suspicion criteria" first mentioned in the DSM-4, which states malingering should be strongly suspected if any of the following factors are noted to be present: (1) medicolegal context of presentation; (2) marked discrepancy between the patient's claimed stress or disability and the objective findings; (3) lack of cooperation during the diagnostic evaluation and in adhering with the prescribed treatment regimen; and (4) the presence of an antisocial personality disorder diagnosis.

Malingering is a deceptive behavior, used opportunistically and episodically. It can involve medical or psychological symptoms and can occur in the presence or absence of psychopathology. Malingering behavior may be enacted for profit, to exploit a situation, or used as a socially acceptable response to adversity. Malingering is not a psychiatric disorder and is considered a nonpathologic condition that may be the focus of clinical attention.[1] Because malingering by itself is not a mental disorder, there are no therapies indicated and no role for inpatient hospitalization to play in its remediation.

Malingering is considered a diagnosis of exclusion, meaning its registration occurs only when the presenting symptoms do not point to an objective etiology. The diagnosis should not be used unless all physical and psychological factors contributing to the patient's presentation have been explored and ruled out. Recently, a large retrospective cross-sectional analysis of emergency department (ED) visits from the National Hospital Ambulatory Medical Care Survey (NHAMCS) data surveying 1,049,695 malingering diagnoses over an 8 year period revealed a malingering prevalence of 0.1% in the ED, which may reflect an appropriate hesitancy by emergency physicians (EPs) to code the diagnosis.[4] Moreover, whites had the highest prevalence and a higher adjusted odds ratio for a malingering diagnosis compared with other races. Another database study sought to determine the prevalence and characteristics of medical malingering in the military, by looking at 28 million health care visits to outpatient settings. During the 6 year study span, clinicians made the diagnosis of malingering in only 985 instances, making the coding of malingering extremely rare.[5]

The true incidence of malingering is unknown, mainly because in most settings it is not possible to know definitively if patients are fabricating or exaggerating symptoms.[6] Some authors have based an estimate upon the registered diagnosis of malingering in the medical records.[4,5,7] This approach may be problematic as malingering is often not coded as a diagnosis, even when suspicion is high.[8] Other authors have simply taken doctors' suspicion of malingering as an actual prevalence which is likely to import the subjective bias of the providers.[9] Suspected malingering is on the rise over the last 20 years, with a 20% baseline rising conspicuously to 42% of patients suspected of malingering at 2 US hospital locations with an emergency psychiatric department over time.[8,9] However, in Europe, the doctors' suspicion of psychiatric malingering is lower with 25% of all patients suspected of simulating to some degree and 8% of patients definitely believed to be simulating.[10] Research efforts show that malingering is very difficult to assess, and coding for it can have far-reaching implications for patients, such as immediate discharge or forgoing admission to the psychiatric hospital.[9]

MALINGERING CASES
Case 1

A 27 year old inmate from the local corrections facility is brought in by EMS for evaluation of self-inflicted injury while on suicide watch. Reportedly, he stood up from his cot and was noted to be covered in blood before passing out briefly in his cell. Emergency medical service (EMS) providers report a minor laceration to the left forearm with nonpulsatile bleeding controlled using direct pressure and estimate blood loss at 1.5 L. Large bore IV access was secured, and 2 L of normal saline was administered in route to the ED. On arrival, he is afebrile, ghostly pale, and diaphoretic, with a pulse of 120 bpm, blood pressure of 90/60, and respirations are 20 with saturations of 95% on room air. Although caked in dried blood, he is conscious and coherent and relates a past medical history of major depressive disorder (MDD) with suicidal ideation (SI) and self-injurious behavior (SIB) and denies being suicidal on self-report. He is on supervised antidepressants and mood stabilizers. This is his third ED visit in the last month for similar injuries. The electronic medical record (EMR) confirms the minor laceration was repaired and lab testing revealed hemoglobin in the 6 to 7.0 g/dL range which led to a prolonged ED stay for blood transfusions. On examination, a 2 cm superficial laceration to the left forearm is noted, distal pulses are intact with full range of motion at the elbow and wrist, and no neurosensory deficits are identified. There is no active bleeding, foreign body or gross contamination at the wound base. He admits the old scars on his extremities were from prior episodes of self-cutting. He asks if a certain EP is working and requests she conduct the laceration repair. Labs are obtained for screening purposes.

Case 2

A 36 year old incarcerated man is brought in by security guards for evaluation of chest pain and palpitations. He has a cardiac history of cocaine-induced myocardial infarction at age 18 years, hypertension and hypercholesterolemia with multiple prior episodes of paroxysmal ventricular tachycardia and MDD with SI in the past. On ED arrival, he states his chest pain is substernal, nonradiating and associated with shortness of breath, intermittent palpitations, and paroxysms of intense pain. He denies any other symptoms, recent cocaine, or other illicit substances and is not taking any prescription medications. He also denies any depressive symptoms or SI. He is afebrile and has stable vital signs with a pulse of 66 beats per minute on monitor, blood pressure of 160/85, respirations of 18, and room air (RA) saturations of 97%. Initial electrocardiogram (EKG) shows normal sinus rhythm (NSR) with a heart rate of 65, and his cardiopulmonary screening examination is within normal limits including a regular heart rate and clear breath sounds noted throughout. About 10 minutes after ED arrival, he develops an episode of ventricular tachycardia (VT) at 220 captured on monitor, lasting less than 10 seconds, during which he clutched his chest with severe pain. His rhythm reverts to NSR at 66 bpm before an EKG can be obtained. He is given 325 mg of aspirin and 2 sublingual nitroglycerin tablets (0.4 mg) which gives him a slight headache. He has several more brief episodes of VT with chest pain. He is given 100 mg lidocaine IV bolus and started on a drip at

1 mg/kg/min and admitted to the CCU for monitoring and continued treatment. Laboratory tests including a negative urine drug screen, electrolytes, troponins, and CBC are within normal limits.

Case 3

A 42 year old woman presents to ED often, complaining of severe lower abdominal pain, 10+ on visual analog scale and "just like when I get a bowel obstruction," with nausea, but no fever, vomiting, diarrhea, or dysuria. She refuses an examination of her abdomen without IV analgesic first, stating "Dilaudid is the only medication that works for my pain." Her EMR lists allergy to non-steroidal anti-inflammatory drugs (NSAIDs) (causing gastrointestinal [GI] distress), and no history of any prior intensive care unit (ICU) admissions. She has a history of MDD without SI and chronic abdominal pain treated with narcotics. Prior surgeries include cholecystectomy last year, total abdominal hysterectomy a few years ago, and appendectomy in childhood. She has had multiple abdominal CT scans. On examination, she is tearful and yelling loudly demanding "Dilaudid now", and she wants the name of the ED doctor in charge. The ED nurse obtains her vital signs which reveal no fever, normal pulse, blood pressure, respiratory rate, and RA saturations. She is notably distressed, but not diaphoretic, or toxic-appearing. She permits an IV start in her right forearm, and after some coaching the ED provider is able to examine her abdomen. Despite the severe tenderness complaint, the abdomen is soft with normally active bowel sounds, no distension or peritoneal signs. She is able to pass flatus and has not vomited at home or while in the ED. She insists on drinking water without staff permission. She refuses to give a urine specimen for analysis. Her other lab tests including electrolytes, complete blood count (CBC), liver function tests, bilirubin, amylase, and lipase are all within normal limits.

Case 4

A 50 year old Hispanic man with the history of end stage renal disease (ESRD) on hemodialysis (HD) is brought in by EMS for evaluation of bleeding from the dialysis needle access site used for connecting up to his arteriovenous (AV) fistula. The bleeding started after leaving the dialysis center. EMS notes brisk bleeding despite the application of direct pressure with gauze and Kerlix. On arrival, the patient is hemodynamically stable and afebrile. The dialysis center is called and confirms that Mr. Z received the full dialysis treatment. They share that he was escorted out of the facility after staffers reported him for using false information to obtain dialysis. He admitted to using his cousin's identification and insurance card when confronted by the clinic manager. Apparently, he is undocumented having arrived illegally from Mexico last week to work in the community. Mr. Z's cousin is well known by providers at the dialysis center and has a history of ESRD on HD complicated by frequent episodes of medical non-adherence with dialysis treatment.

DIFFERENTIAL DIAGNOSIS FOR MALINGERED SOMATIC SYMPTOMS

EPs employ a traditional diagnostic approach—obtaining a detailed history, conducting a physical examination, and ordering ancillary studies (lab, imaging) in constructing a differential diagnosis of probable illness. When they find this approach insufficient to explain a patient's symptoms, EPs must reconsider the presentation features and other elements to broaden their differential diagnostic framework. This retracement may allow the EP to parse other possibilities to explain the patient's symptoms and is especially useful when faced with exaggerated signs or symptoms that seem suspicious. When possible organic etiologies do not align with objective findings in the ED workup and are excluded from diagnostic consideration, the potential for the patient's "disease" including concerns for psychological, somatic symptoms disorders, and malingering arises.

The intersection between organic and inorganic symptoms is integral to the differential diagnosis of a potentially malingering patient. A patient presenting to the ED with a seemingly organic chief complaint can actually be masking a somatic, or psychologically driven, symptom. Conversely, a seemingly somatic symptom can be masking an underlying organic pathology.

Organic symptoms themselves have had a long history of complex and misunderstood presentations. For instance, before the discovery of *Helicobacter pylori*, many infected patients were diagnosed with gastric ulcers of unknown etiology and not treated with curative antibiotics. Organic diseases commonly mistaken for those with somatic origins include endocrine disorders (thyroid disorders, Addison disease, insulinoma), poisoning (botulism, carbon monoxide), hereditary metabolic disorders (Wilson disease, homocystinuria, Niemann–Pick disease type C), multiple sclerosis, myasthenia gravis, and systemic lupus erythematosus.[11–18] These "madness mimickers" can complicate the EP's task of filtering malingered symptoms from those with underlying organic or somatic components, particularly those which pose an acute threat to the patient.[11]

Conversely, patients with inorganic symptoms may present with what seems like an acute, organic symptom. For instance, a patient may present with acute chest or abdominal pain. With severe physical symptoms, the EP should always address the chief complaint. The medical history, physical examination, and diagnostic testing may be helpful to rule out organic disease. It is important to engage the patient and inform them promptly of the results in the shared medical decision-making process. It is only when this traditional approach returns nondiagnostic results, that the EP must consider underlying possible somatic explanation or malingering. A medical screening examination (MSE) under US law is mandated for every patient that comes to the ED to rule out an acute emergency medical condition. Eliciting the goals and values of the patient throughout the ED visit is important in the shared decision-making process. Certainly, pure somatic symptoms, conversion, and other psychiatric disorders do present to the ED and require a careful approach to detect.

Once an organic origin of the patient's signs and symptoms has been ruled out, the EP should use the differential diagnosis outlined in **Fig. 1**.[19] In this framework, the first judgment involves whether the patient's complaint is an intentional act of deception. If so, then the EP should carefully discern whether the deception is motivated by an external incentive. This includes avoiding work, gaining hospital admission, getting out of jail, or obtaining prescription medications. If so, the patient is likely malingering. If not, then the patient may have a factitious disorder. This is the only other psychiatric disorder of the 70 listed in the DSM-5 in which the patient *intentionally* falsifies medical or psychiatric symptoms on themselves or upon another, either self-induced or fabricated, purely for internal gains, or are motivated by inner compulsion.[1,20] Previously, Munchausen's disorder and Munchausen's by proxy were descriptions for factitious disorder where symptoms are directed toward one's self or upon another, respectively. If intentional deception by the patient has been ruled out, the EP should ascertain whether the patient may be feigning voluntary motor or sensory dysfunction such as sudden blindness, numbness, paralysis, or seizures but without an underlying neurologic basis. This combination describes a functional diagnosis most consistent with conversion disorder. If a conversion disorder has been ruled out, then the EP

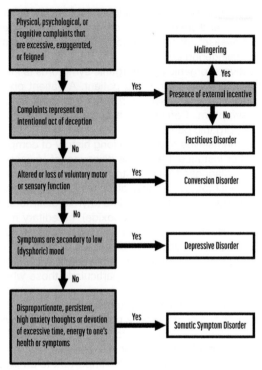

Fig. 1. A differential diagnosis to guide EPs to discern malingering patients from those with psychiatric or somatic symptom disorders.[19]

should judge whether the symptoms are secondary to a dysphoric mood. Somatic symptom disorder is characterized by incessant thoughts or persistently high anxiety regarding their health and/or symptoms, which causes a disruption of their ability to function in everyday life. The patient's symptoms feel very real to them. Often these patients cannot be convinced that the clinical testing results are normal and fail to be reassured by the EP's assessment of the derived findings.

If the EP's differential diagnosis has reached this final tier in **Fig. 1**, then it likely involves another, more complex factor. Up to 67% of patients with somatic symptom disorders also present with a personality disorder.[21] Personality disorders can be grouped into 3 presentation styles—cluster A, B, and C personality disorders. These clusters and the recommended interpersonal approach to best facilitate each type's ED care are described in **Fig. 2**. Cluster A personality disorders are characterized by quiet, paranoid, cautious personality traits, and strange or unusual behaviors. Cluster A patients should be treated with curiosity and a direct conversational style. Medical conversations should be concise and easily accessible to the patient. Cluster B personality disorders are characterized by loudness, fragility, drug-seeking, suicidal tendencies, and a demanding or antisocial personality. If cluster B traits are identified, the EP should set firm boundaries and employ an abundantly calm, conversational style. Cluster C personality disorders are characterized by nervousness, indecisiveness, inflexibility, and poor coping strategies. Should these traits be identified, the EP should be calm and direct. In all instances, the provider should maintain a safe distance, voice, and message that stays: Neutral, Empathetic, and Avoids Labeling (NEAL). If these personality disorders are known and not factored into ED workup,

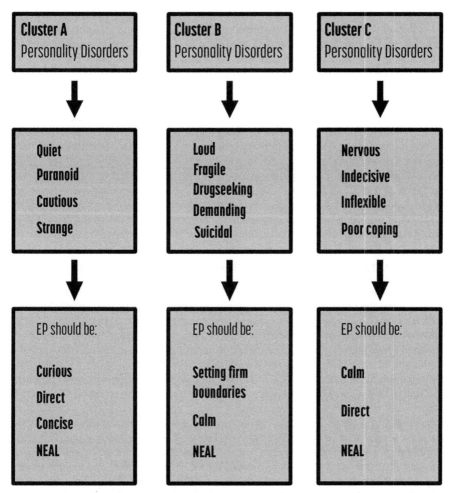

Fig. 2. A characterization of key traits for patients with clusters A, B, and C personality disorders. Additionally, it describes specific conversational styles with which the EP should treat patients with these personality disorders. NEAL: neutral, empathetic, avoid labeling.

early on, the patient may become less interactive or aggressive when the provider poses questions. Alternatively, the unprepared provider may become frustrated and abandon further inquiry, leaving a potential somatic symptom disorder unidentified which may be more amenable to primary care follow-up and treatment than the personality disorder.

Additional information found in the patient's EMR may be helpful. Although psychiatry notes may be protected from viewing, diagnosed conditions and disorders are often curated and listed under past medical history. These data may be very helpful in sorting out prior visits and have possible relevance to the current presentation. The EMR can reveal patterns of drug-seeking behavior, substance misuse, feigned symptoms, or other suspicious presentations that may be attributable to malingering. Determining that a patient is acting in bad faith is difficult, especially because encounters tend to be handled as isolated, unique visits and providers may be unfamiliar with a patient's pattern of behavior. However, increasingly with the advent of EMRs detecting evidence of behavior patterns, previous ED visits, logged laboratory results, and comparative imaging have become easier to access and analyze. Moreover, screening for ED recidivism patterns, baseline lab values, imaging frequency, and results can be helpful in supplying clinical truth when negotiating with patients concerned with illness possibilities during the ED visit.

Once malingering is suspected, it is important for the EP to consider their role in the greater context of the health care system. Quite simply, the EP must first exclude life or limb threatening diagnoses, stabilize and evaluate the patient for admission, or transfer the patient to another hospital for ongoing treatment. The EP is not responsible for labeling the patient as a malingerer or for making a new diagnosis of personality, nonsuicidal psychiatric, or somatic symptom disorders. The EP should not let the suspicion of malingering dissolve established rapport with the patient. Instead, they should use this suspicion to optimize patient outcomes. When these diagnoses are suspected, patients can be safely discharged to their primary care physician (PCP) for close follow-up. Together, they can consider broadening the medical differential or fielding subspecialty referral for psychiatry or pain clinic management as appropriate.

ETHICAL CONSIDERATIONS ARISING WHEN MALINGERING IS SUSPECTED

Our case scenarios highlight the ethical dilemmas that arise in the doctor–patient relationship when the patient engages in malingering behavior. There is a paucity of documented cases of malingering in the medical ethics literature that makes it unclear at what point the rights of a patient and the obligations of the provider break down when a patient is acting in bad faith.[22,23] Ethical discussions in emergency medicine usually assume that health care providers have an obligation to help their patients, but patients are also assumed to be seeking care with honest intentions. Questioning health care provider obligations, even when a patient's intentions are not honest, can lead to providers being viewed as dismissive or even abusive. Health care providers who question their responsibility to patients' risk being viewed in a negative light. Although ethical principles in medicine strive to improve patient care and the health of the public by examining and promoting physician professionalism, some of these principles can be difficult if not impossible to apply when patients are manipulative and do not act in good faith. Examining the medical ethics concepts of patient autonomy, beneficence, nonmaleficence, and justice, and elucidating how these concepts should be adapted when the patients do not act in good faith is the goal of the next section.

Autonomy

The concept of patient autonomy holds that a competent person is at liberty to decide what shall and shall not be done therapeutically to their own body.[24] The individual may consent to treatment, refuse specific treatments or drugs, and may sign out against medical advice. Although a patient has every right to ask his or her health care provider for a specific treatment, the health care provider is not required to yield to the patient's requests—or demands—for a "therapy" that is known to be nonbeneficial or even harmful (eg, Case 3 opioids for a patient with chronic pain) or to dictate unreasonable (dangerous and expensive) interventions (Cases 2 and 4). Providers should respect the rights of patients to make medical decisions that reflect their own goals and values. Decisions should be based on clear and accurate information and should be free of coercion. Every effort should be made to come to a mutually agreeable course of action to diagnose and treat the patient's condition. If an accord cannot be struck, the physician is under no obligation to provide care that is contrary to their professional judgment or moral beliefs.[25]

Beneficence

The concept of beneficence indicates there is a provider obligation to act in the best interests of patients and applies to all case scenarios. The provider has a duty to do good and promote the patient's welfare. EPs are obliged, especially, to rescue a patient with diminished capacity at risk of harm.[24] This idea is the basis for admission for SI. In Case 1, the patient's lack of SI notwithstanding, the life-threatening hemorrhage due to SIB enables the patient to repeatedly manipulate the system. The doctor–patient relationship should be a 2-way obligation, but it frequently is defined as rights of the patient (eg, access to medical care) and as obligations for the doctor. Deception and abuse of the doctor by the patient, when portrayed as unthinkable by ethicists, results in no societal plan of action for those who would abuse health care rights. As in all shared decision-making, the doctor should recommend the best diagnostic and treatment regimen and have a discussion with the patient about risks, benefits, and how this fits with the patient's goals and values.

Nonmaleficence

The concept of nonmaleficence is closely entwined with beneficence but serves to emphasize "first do no harm." This rule applies in an active sense; for example, not prescribing opioids to a patient with chronic pain (Case 3). Adherence to this rule can put the provider in direct conflict (and harm's way) with some patients, such as disingenuous drug-seeking malingerers (Case 2) and the disorderly chronic pain professors (Case 3). Nevertheless, providers are in accord with this rule when they avoid creating risk for a patient through inaction. Therefore, providers are ethically obligated to take every threat of suicide seriously, even if the word 'suicide' is denied. Although the physician may feel manipulated by the patient's actions (Case 1), the physician may objectively determine the need for transfusion and gauge the threat of self-harm. Also the duty to avoid harm supports not repeating CT scans to avoid unnecessary radiation and associated costs without a clinical indication (Case 3).

Justice

Justice aligns a duty to apply fairness in processes and distribution of benefits at a macro level. This applies in all the case scenarios. Justice considerations include 3 broad categories: respect for patient rights, distribution of scarce resources, and abiding with morally acceptable laws crafted by society. Some medical interventions may be expensive and labor or resource intensive. Deploying such interventions should be carefully considered by the medical community to ensure their appropriate use.[26] In general, the high cost of a specific treatment (eg, HD) should not influence the care of an individual patient if proven to be efficacious. However, there are times stewardship of resources, when federally granted, requires acting on the boundary lines (Case 4). There is a need to define a proper balance between societal and professional beneficence and freeloading behavior. Demonstrations of bad faith by patients may get them "fired" from the private practices of the institution, but the safety net function of the hospital ED, without exception, is to be available always and to all persons arriving for evaluation.

EXISTING LAWS TO UPHOLD ETHICAL CONSIDERATIONS
EMTALA

Emergency Medical Treatment and Active Labor Act (EMTALA) applies to all the case scenarios. EMTALA became US Law in 1986 to formally address the problem of patient dumping; previously private hospitals were in the practice of briefly seeing and registering patients (hospital ID bands placed) and then sending them away to public hospitals because they were deemed to be unable to pay for emergency services (destitute, uninsured, underinsured).

EMTALA ensures that all patients with a medical emergency will be treated at any hospital to which they present or be transferred safely to one that can manage their care. Specifically, anyone who presents to a hospital is entitled to a MSE by a qualified medical provider (QMP) to determine whether an emergency medical condition or active labor is present. An emergency medical condition is defined as any acute illness that left untreated would result in serious damage to the health of the patient or unborn baby. If such a condition is present, medical stabilization must be provided regardless of the patient's ability to pay for it. Such stabilization includes any evaluation and treatment necessary to ensure that the patient's condition will not deteriorate when discharged. This may require inpatient hospitalization. If the hospital is unable to provide the services a patient needs, the hospital must make the patient stable for transport and arrange transfer to another hospital that can provide those services. A hospital with the available resources to treat a patient cannot refuse a transfer from another hospital that lacks those resources. QMP involved in providing MSE and evaluation with stabilization for transfer if need be include physicians, physician assistants, nurse practitioners, and midwives.

With the advent of EMTALA, hospitals' participation in and reimbursement by Medicare became tied to their compliance with EMTALA rules. Hospitals that violate EMTALA risk getting dropped from Medicare. Each EMTALA violation carries a significant monetary penalty of $50,000 for both the doctor at fault and the hospital itself. Furthermore, EMTALA applies not only to emergency providers who manage the initial treatment of patients, but also to any consultants who are needed to help stabilize and admit patients.

Health Insurance Portability and Accountability Act

The Health Insurance Portability and Accountability Act (HIPAA) Privacy Rule does not address medical identity theft directly; it does describe in detail the uses and disclosures of personal health information (PHI) that are permitted without formal authorization from patients. These include for the "purpose of treatment, payment, and healthcare operations activities" and "incident to an otherwise permitted use and disclosure." This would allow for reporting identity theft to the authorities (Case 4). However, the HIPAA Privacy Rule also states that providers (covered entities) should "rely on professional ethics and best judgments in deciding which of these permissive uses and disclosures to make." Thus, although the HIPAA Privacy Rule may technically allow sharing of PHI under the circumstances, the rule itself compels us to be judicious and conscious of our professional obligation to act in the patient's best interest, as we make choices about how and when to disclose information. In regard to Case 4, we must rely on our professional ethical compass to help us make decisions that balance the often competing duties and responsibilities that we carry as emergency medicine physicians. In fact, Case 4 is an example of a real imposter, an individual who impersonates another to take scarce resources that they are not entitled to receive. Twice Mr. Z has attempted to register under his cousin's name for the delivery of medical services. Some may argue that since he presented with a post-dialysis complication, the medical system owes him complementary treatment, whoever he truly is. Under EMTALA, we can find our purpose in exercising a moral duty that pertains to beneficence and acting on the legal mandate to provide an MSE in the ED and to render any medically necessary stabilizing treatment. However, some authors go further[27] and fail to see the seriousness of suspected medical identity theft. They claim it is an HIPAA breach to report such activities and that ethically and legally there is no duty to report a crime. Although the latter may be true, the former is clearly wrong. HIPAA should not be used to keep the secrets of imposters hidden.

RED FLAG RULES, 2008 AND CLARIFICATION 2010

In 2008, the Federal Trade Commission issued regulations known as the Red Flag Rules, which required hospital institutions to develop and implement written identity theft prevention programs.[28] Congress later passed the Red Flag Clarification Act of 2010, which eased the requirements, thereby allowing many health care organizations to be exempt from this regulation. Consequently, many hospital institutions have not instituted policies on medical identity theft or provided physician or nonphysician staff the needed skills to counteract this type of fraud.

Medical identity theft in the ED can harm numerous individuals, and many frontline health care providers are unaware of this growing concern. There have been cases discovered in ED encounters where red flags were discovered by registration clerks upon validating the patient's identity and discrepancies were shared with physicians. These reported incidents were handled without compromising patient care or EMTALA regulations.[29] Educating all health care personnel within and outside the ED regarding the subtle signs of medical identity theft and implementing institutional policies to identify these criminals may discourage further fraudulent behavior.[22] Real imposters have been charged with suspected medical identity theft and later convicted of felony for medical identity theft and insurance fraud.[29]

RESOLUTION OF CASES
Case 1

A 27 year old inmate denies suicidal intent of his SIB. He states he is bored with being confined on suicide watch, and impulsively cut his arm at the same spot as before with "a tough toenail, to feel better." He has been taking supervised psychiatric medications that aren't helping him to manage his self-harm urges and counseling services available to him are very limited. He wants to be transferred to another prison. He has concluded the easiest way to accomplish this is to make himself a nuisance for the jailers, so "they want to get rid of me." The laceration is repaired. Labs reveal a hemoglobin value of 6.5 g/dL. Given his low blood pressures and tachycardia after the initial fluid bolus, he is given a 2-unit blood transfusion. He is discharged back to prison in police custody with strict instructions for close behavioral surveillance and given a recommendation for additional psychiatric counseling. His diagnoses also include the new symptomatic codes from the DSM-5-TR which identifies *suicidal and non-suicidal self-injurious behaviors.*[3] Future clinicians now have a systematic way to track prevalence of these behaviors and other correlating factors that need ongoing attention.

Case 2

A 36 year old incarcerated man admitted to the cardiac care unit (CCU) for ongoing chest pain with paroxysmal ventricular tachycardia on a lidocaine infusion for an hour. After multiple recurrences of the dysrhythmia in the CCU, one episode of tachycardia was finally captured on a 12-lead EKG. Notably, the appearance of a wide-complex tachyarrhythmia was confined to lead V3, during which time all other leads demonstrated NSR. This finding was inconsistent with VT and could only be explained as motion artifact.[23] On closer observation, the patient was witnessed to be tapping on the lead V3 sensor patch repeatedly. When confronted, the patient confessed to intentionally tapping on the lead to simulate cardiac dysrhythmia. He gave no reason for doing this. Eventually medical records became available and showed the patient had similar previous CCU admissions, all occurring without capture of an EKG during his ongoing period of incarceration and none documenting a diagnosis of malingering. In this case, malingering was proven in the CCU so coding the diagnosis of malingering is important. By malingering in this way the patient has subjected himself to potentially dangerous interventions, and inflicted a significant cost to society. Perhaps the source of external gain was the temporary reprieve from prison or drug seeking behavior. As ethical physicians we want to limit the harm from unnecessary cardiac medications and interventions and begin psychiatric interventions that may be beneficial.[23]

Case 3

A 42 year old woman complaining of severe abdominal pain, who has specific requests for Dilaudid, repeated imaging with a history of chronic abdominal pain that appears unresolved by prior abdominal surgery. This is a difficult case because of the loud and demanding nature of her presentation. She seems to be overtly seeking drugs and may have a somatic symptom disorder. In addition, she struggles with normal daily activities, which are punctuated by the high frequency of her ED visits. Her self-reported history of no vomiting, fever, or any features typical of bowel obstruction makes the presentation even more suspicious. Given the discordant history and unimpressive examination, the question becomes one of discovering the goals of therapy from the patient's perspective. As doctors make efforts to meet the patient in the middle, understanding shared expectations can be crucial for medical decision-making that is acceptable to both. Communicating with this patient in a neutral, empathetic fashion (NEAL) that avoids labeling her pain as out of proportion or exaggerated may help the clinical interaction. On the one hand, EPs have a duty, dictated by the ethical principle of beneficence, to treat patients with respect and dignity within the context of the doctor–patient relationship. The appropriate and adequate treatment of pain in the ED is an EP's duty within this relationship. On the other hand, providing medications to a patient in the acute setting of the ED that might exacerbate an underlying illness of addiction and dependence is concerning and may cause more harm than good. Similarly, obtaining expensive CT imaging to confirm the expected, clinically normal findings simply because the patient has come to expect this at the ED is not ideal either. Ultimately, the EP has the autonomy to make treatment decisions based on a clinical judgment about what will be beneficial or harmful to the patient. If in the shared decision-making process there is no agreement reached, the physician should offer the tests and therapies that promote the most good (health and well-being) to the patient. In this case and as always, unnecessary, expensive, or potentially harmful interventions should not go forward, even when the patient demands it. The diagnosis of abdominal pain, chronic and somatic symptom disorder is appropriate. She is told to follow up with her PCP for referral to a pain specialist and possibly a psychiatrist to help devise coping strategies for her chronic pain.

Case 4

Under EMTALA, a medical screening examination to rule out life or limb threats is performed by the doctor. Mr. Z complains of bleeding from the needle site used to access the fistula earlier in the day at the dialysis center. He is not on any blood thinners and denies any trauma to the arm since leaving dialysis. On examination he looks chronically ill, but not toxic. His right upper extremity is bleeding venous blood a few inches from the AV fistula. Palpation of the fistula reveals a strong thrill and auscultation confirms an audible bruit. Distal pulses are intact. Brisk nonpulsatile bleeding is noted from the skin puncture site, when direct pressure is removed. After consent is obtained a single 3-0 nylon suture in a figure 8 pattern is placed superficially at the puncture site. Upon discharge, the patient again uses his cousin's identification and insurance card for ED visit billing. The registration clerk notifies the ED manager of the situation and they call the local authorities to investigate Mr. Z for suspicion of medical identity theft. After a police report is filed, Mr. Z is discharged from the ED with a diagnosis of post HD bleeding complication and ESRD on HD.

Medical identity theft is a crime and if convicted Mr. Z could be charged with a felony. Similar to malingerers, who may waste medical resources, he can be charged with theft of services.[22,23,30] Real imposters that don't pay their bills may be charged with theft of services if hospitals or the impersonated patients press charges.

Finally, it should be mentioned that in the case of Mr. Z the health providers that are "covered entities" under the HIPAA are entitled to report crimes under 45 CFR 164.512(f) (5): "A covered entity may disclose to a law enforcement official protected health information that the covered entity believes in good faith constitutes evidence of criminal conduct that occurred on the premises of the covered entity".[31,32]

SUMMARY

Assessing, identifying, and handling a malingering patient can be quite a challenge for providers, especially without the help of effective management strategies. As demonstrated by the variety in our series of malingering case presentations, providers must be mindful of the complexities of serving frustrating patients. There are many medical disorders that rely on patient self-reporting of pain or anxiety that may lack objective clinical parameters. These symptoms can be exaggerated to obtain medications, e.g. sickle cell anemia, chronic pancreatitis, and seizures. Still, it is critical to avoid judging patients and preserve an open channel of communication. Malingering should be thought of as a call for aid. This call is best answered by EPs when they apply our NEAL strategy. EPs are encouraged to engage the patient in shared medical decision-making throughout their ED visit, and to secure PCP follow-up of their concerns. In most instances, it is not recommended that providers confront the patient or register the diagnosis of malingering in the ED because the downstream effects of this label can also malinger.

CLINICS CARE POINTS

- Difficult patients may present with a mix of psychiatric and physical issues, and may be categorized as malingerers, true feigners, chronic complainers, and/or real imposters.

- Malingering is a diagnosis of exclusion that involves the intentional simulation or significant exaggeration of symptoms.

- ED management includes remaining NEAL to optimize outcomes for shared medical decision-making.

DISCLOSURE

Authors have no conflict of interest to declare.

REFERENCES

1. American Psychiatric Association. Diagnostic and statistical manual of mental disorders. 5th ed. Washington, D.C.: American Psychiatric Publication; 2013.
2. ICD-11 for mortality and morbidity statistics. 2019. Available at: https://icd.who.int/browse11/1-m/en#/http://id.who.int/icd/entity/1136473465. Accessed 22 Nov 2022.
3. American Psychiatric Association. Diagnostic and statistical manual of mental disorders. 5th ed. Washington, D.C.: American Psychiatric Publishing Inc.; 2022. Revised.
4. Udoetuk S, Dongarwar D, Salihu HM. Racial and gender disparities in diagnosis of malingering in clinical settings. J Racial Ethn Health Disparities 2020;7(6): 1117–23.
5. Lande RG, Williams LB. Prevalence and characteristics of military malingering. Mil Med 2013;178(1):50–4.
6. Gudjonsson G., Detection strategies for malingering and defensiveness, In: Rogers R., Clinical assessment of malingering and deception, 3rd edition, Guilford Press; New York, 14–35.
7. Park L, Costello S, Li J, et al. Race, health, and socioeconomic disparities associated with malingering in psychiatric patients at an urban emergency department. Gen Hosp Psychiatry 2021;71:121–7.
8. Yates BD, Nordquist CR, Schultz-Ross RA. Feigned psychiatric symptoms in the emergency room. Psychiatr Serv 1996;47(9):998–1000.
9. Rumschik SM, Appel JM. Malingering in the psychiatric emergency department: prevalence, predictors, and outcomes. Psychiatr Serv 2019;70(2):115–22.
10. Boberg M, Jeppesen U, Arnfred S, et al. Do we know the mind of others? Suspicion of malingering in emergency psychiatry. Nord J Psychiatry 2022;1–6. https://doi.org/10.1080/08039488.2022.2083676, published online ahead of print, 2022 Jun 17.
11. Moukaddam N, AufderHeide E, Flores A, et al. Shift, interrupted: strategies for managing difficult patients including those with personality disorders and somatic symptoms in the emergency department. Emerg Med Clin North Am 2015;33(4):797–810.
12. Demily C, Sedel F. Psychiatric manifestations of treatable hereditary metabolic disorders in adults. Ann Gen Psychiatry 2014;13:27.
13. Min YW, Rhee PL. Noncardiac chest pain: update on the diagnosis and management. Korean J Gastroenterol 2015;65(2):76–84.
14. Fass R, Achem SR. Noncardiac chest pain: epidemiology, natural course and pathogenesis. J Neurogastroenterol Motil 2011;17(2):110–23.
15. Krarup AL, Liao D, Gregersen H, et al. Nonspecific motility disorders, irritable esophagus, and chest pain. Ann N Y Acad Sci 2013;1300:96–109.
16. Fass R, Navarro-Rodriguez T. Noncardiac chest pain. J Clin Gastroenterol 2008; 42(5):636–46.
17. Coss-Adame E, Erdogan A, Rao SS. Treatment of esophageal (noncardiac) chest pain: an expert review. Clin Gastroenterol Hepatol 2014;12(8):1224–45, published correction appears in Clin Gastroenterol Hepatol. 2015 May;13(5):1031.
18. Macalpine I, Hunter R. The 'insanity of King George III': a classic case of porphyria. Br Med J 1966;1(5479):65–71.
19. Martin PK, Schroeder RW. Challenges in assessing and managing malingering, factitious disorder, and related somatic disorder. Psychiatr Times 2014;32(10):19.

20. Carnahan KT, Jha A. Factitious disorder. Treasure Island (FL): StatPearls Publishing; 2022. StatPearls.
21. Garcia-Campayo J, Alda M, Sobradiel N, et al. Personality disorders in somatization disorder patients: a controlled study in Spain. J Psychosom Res 2007;62(6): 675–80.
22. Huynh R, Thoms A, Nguyen TM, et al. The missing spleen - A diagnosis of medical identity fraud in surgery: Case report. Int J Surg Case Rep 2021;78:210–3.
23. Kefalas S, Ezenkwele U. Wide-complex tachycardia as the presenting complaint in a case of malingering. J Emerg Med 2006;30(2):159–61.
24. Beauchamp TL, Childress JF. Principles of biomedical ethics. 6th ed. New York, NY: Oxford University Press; 2008.
25. American College of Emergency Physicians. Nonbeneficial ("futile") emergency medical intervention. Revised 2017b. Available at: https://www.acep.org/patient-care/policy-statements/nonbeneficial-futile-emergency-medical-interventions/. Accessed January 2, 2023.
26. American College of Emergency Physicians. Emergency physicians stewardship of finite resources. Revised 2019. Available at: https://www.acep.org/patient-care/policy-statements/emergency-physician-stewardship-of-finite-resources/. Accessed December 21, 2022.
27. Gorgas DL, Li-Sauerwine S. No country for sick men: Undocumented persons. In: Baker EF, editor. Legal and ethical issues in emergency medicine, what do i do now emergency medicine. New York: Oxford Academic; 2020. p. 83–7.
28. Alexander J. Healthcare organizations must have an identity theft policy: FACTA or FICTION? Healthc Financ Manage 2008;62(9):38–40.
29. Mancini M. Medical identity theft in the emergency department: awareness is crucial. West J Emerg Med 2014;15(7):899–901.
30. Appel JM. From malingering to theft of service. Am Acad Psychiatry Law Newsletter 2016;8:24.
31. US Department of Health and Human Services, Office for Civil Rights, Standards for privacy of individually identifiable health information; security standards for the protection of electronic protected health information; general administrative requirements including civil monetary penalties; procedures for investigations, imposition of penalties, and hearings. Regulation text, 45 CFR Parts 160 and 164. December 28, 2000 as amended: May 31, 2002, August 14, 2002, February 20, 2003 and April 17, 2003.
32. 45 C.F.R. § 164.512 (2003): Uses and disclosures for which an authorization or opportunity to agree or object is not required. See § 164.512(f)(5).

Legal and Ethical Considerations in Psychiatric Emergencies

Jay M. Brenner, MD[a],*, Thomas E. Robey, MD, PhD[b]

KEYWORDS

• Individual rights • Custody • Malingering

KEY POINTS

• Individual rights can be limited in the context of psychiatric emergencies.
• Mental health emergencies present unique dilemmas of care and disposition that are informed by both standard of care and local statute.
• Patients in custody present alternative options for disposition from the emergency department.

INTRODUCTION

This article addresses legal and ethical considerations in the practice of emergency medicine. Allen and colleagues[1] ably considered capacity and consent, privacy and confidentiality, and involuntary treatment. The authors consider a patient presenting to the emergency department (ED) with depression and suicidality, a patient with psychosis and homicidal ideation, and a patient with anxiety and malingering, to further examine patient rights, in-custody issues, and what to do when it appears a patient is attempting to escape a trial appearance.

Mental health statutes vary widely in their scope and application. In addition to other sections of this issue, the reader is advised to refer to state medical associations for guidance with regard to specific practice surrounding individuals' rights in the context of custody issues or incapacity during mental health emergencies. The general discussion offered in this article is offered as a foundation for reviewing similar situations in American emergency medicine practice.

The authors have no conflicts of interest to disclose.

[a] SUNY–Upstate Medical University, 750 East Adams Street, Syracuse, NY 13210, USA; [b] Elson S. Floyd College of Medicine, Washington State University, Providence Regional Medical Center Everett, 1700 13th Street, Everett, WA 98201, USA

* Corresponding author.

E-mail address: brennerj@upstate.edu

CASE 1

An 18-year-old woman presents to the ED complaining of suicidal ideations after overdosing on pills. She is medically cleared, seen by the psychiatry consultation service, and deemed to require an admission. She is willing to sign a voluntary application; however, there are no beds available. She remains a boarder in the ED awaiting psychiatric bed placement. What rights does she have?

PATIENT RIGHTS

Patients who present to the ED with suicidality are entitled to a medical screening and mental health screening process that protects their human dignity while balancing their autonomy with the beneficence of caring for them. Emergency physicians (EPs) and other providers also must observe the duty to follow laws applicable to self-harm.

Autonomy

A competent patient with decision-making capacity has the autonomy to make their own health care decisions unless they are deemed a risk to themselves or others. A patient who expresses current suicidality is a risk to themselves, and it is therefore a right of the physician to overrule their autonomy for the patient's benefit. Many states distinguish between voluntary and involuntary placements in a conditional manner. Patients may volunteer to be admitted for treatment without activating statutes of involuntary holds, but occasionally patients at risk of self-harm may change their minds in the same visit and then are no longer voluntary. At this point, the legal mechanisms of detainment are activated.

Physician-Patient Relationship

An EP cannot override a patient's autonomy until they have a relationship with the patient. This relationship is established upon arrival to the ED.

Obtaining Nonconsensual Collateral Information

HIPAA expressly permits collateral information to be obtained without patient consent.[2] In *Jablonski v United States*, a psychiatrist was held liable for not doing so.[3] Although HIPAA does not explicitly discuss reviewing publicly available information, an EP may obtain patient information that is publicly available. Data sources may include court dockets, news sources, social media, mapping software, employment-related content, videos, and photographs. Suicide notes can include text messages, e-mails, or social media posts.[4]

Medical Screening

The American College of Emergency Physicians (ACEP) clinical policy offers recommendations with regard to medical screening (**Table 1**).[5] This includes recommendations for laboratories and especially the role of urine drug screens and blood-ethanol levels.

Voluntary Hospitalization

A great way to enhance a patient's sense of autonomy is to offer voluntary hospitalization to competent patients who have decision-making capacity. The American Psychiatric Association Task Force on Consent to Voluntary Hospitalization recognizes the many advantages of a voluntary admission over an involuntary admission. It maintains the patient's autonomy, maximizes the patient's rights, reduces stigma, broadens access to inpatient care as many patients do not meet the criteria for involuntary

Table 1
American College of Emergency Physicians recommendations for medical screening

Patient Management Recommendations	Level A	Level B	Level C
What testing is necessary in order to determine medical stability in alert, cooperative patients with normal vital signs, a noncontributory history and physical examination, and psychiatric symptoms?	None specified	In adult ED patients with primary psychiatric complaints, diagnostic evaluation should be directed by the history and physical examination. Routine laboratory testing of all patients is of very low yield and need not be performed as part of the ED assessment	None specified
Do the results of a urine drug screen for drugs of abuse affect management in alert, cooperative patients with normal vital signs, a noncontributory history and physical examination, and a psychiatric complaint?	None specified	None specified	1. Routine urine toxicologic screens for drugs of abuse in alert, awake, cooperative patients do not affect ED management and need not be performed as part of the ED assessment 2. Urine toxicologic screens for drugs of abuse obtained in the ED for the use of the receiving psychiatric facility or service should not delay patient evaluation or transfer
Does an elevated alcohol level preclude the initiation of a psychiatric evaluation in alert, cooperative patients with normal vital signs and a noncontributory history and physical examination?	None specified	None specified	1. The patient's cognitive abilities, rather than a specific blood-alcohol level, should be the basis on which clinicians begin the psychiatric assessment 2. Consider using a period of observation to determine if psychiatric symptoms resolve as the episode of intoxication resolves

Lukens, TW et al. "Clinical Policy: Critical Issues in the Diagnosis and Management of the Adult Psychiatric Patient in the Emergency Department." Annals of Emergency Medicine. Vol. 47. No. 1. Pages 79 to 99. January 2006.

admission, may allow for earlier treatment initiation before patients are more deteriorated, enhances the collaborative treatment relationship, may lead to more favorable outcome, and avoids increased costs for the mental health system and the courts that are incurred by involuntary admission processes.[6]

(In-)Justice of Scarce Resources

With mental health resources taxed beyond capacity in most jurisdictions, the contrast between ideal treatment and the typical practice is stark. Although a patient seeking help for an emergency presentation with suicidal thoughts should receive prompt clearance, expedient mental health evaluation, and straight-forward behavioral health admission, they typically experience days of emergency boarding until definitive care is arranged. It is not surprising that this suboptimal care could lead to voluntary decisions for hospitalization to escalate to involuntary interventions. Health systems everywhere are faced with the scarce resources of mental health practitioners and inpatient behavioral health beds, leaving EDs to aspire to provide the most humane care within circumstances that challenge privacy and mental health standard of care, and statutes (such as a 72-hour hold) requiring expedient care.

CASE 2

A 36-year-old man in police custody presents to the ED complaining of demonic voices telling him to strip naked and run down city streets and loot stores while attacking anyone in his way. He is medically cleared with the exception of screening positive for cannabinoids. The psychiatry consultation service recommends involuntary admission. An alternative option offered by law enforcement is that he be brought to jail, where he may receive psychiatric care via telemedicine. What should you do?

IN-CUSTODY ISSUES

Patients brought into the ED in custody have limited rights because of either being incarcerated or being under arrest. They may have further infringements on their rights if they are deemed a risk to themselves or others. Incarcerated patients may have in-person or remote psychiatry care available to them in prison; however, patients who are in custody pending arraignment may have limited access to such services. Nonetheless, law enforcement officials have jurisdiction over a patient's disposition if that disposition is prison or jail once medical screening is complete. If the patient is going to receive only a ticket for an appearance in court rather than being brought to jail, then the patient may receive mental health care in the hospital. Of course, it is possible that the patient who is acutely psychotic may become agitated when the EP recommends admission and require additional medical intervention.

Humane Agitation Management

When a patient is agitated, an EP can attempt verbal de-escalation. If this fails, chemical and even mechanical restraint may become necessary to protect the patient and staff from injury. Every effort should be made, however, to limit the power differential between the EP and patient in order to preserve the therapeutic relationship. Here is some specific guidance that may help to do this while in the ED.

- Clearly communicate that interventions are "for protection and prevention, and not punishment."
- Minimize confrontation with communication that intends to save face for all parties.

Table 2
American College of Emergency Physicians recommendations for sedation

Patient Management Recommendations	Level A	Level B	Level C
What is the most effective pharmacologic treatment for the acutely agitated patient in the ED?	None specified	1. Use a benzodiazepine (lorazepam or midazolam) or a conventional antipsychotic (droperidol or haloperidol) as effective monotherapy for the initial drug treatment of the acutely agitated undifferentiated patient in the ED 2. If rapid sedation is required, consider droperidol instead of haloperidol 3. Use an antipsychotic (typical or atypical) as effective monotherapy for both management of agitation and initial drug therapy for the patient with known psychiatric illness for which antipsychotics are indicated 4. Use a combination of an oral benzodiazepine (lorazepam) and an oral antipsychotic (risperidone) for agitated but cooperative patients	The combination of a parenteral benzodiazepine and haloperidol may produce more rapid sedation than monotherapy in the acutely agitated psychiatric patient in the ED

Lukens, TW et al. "Clinical Policy: Critical Issues in the Diagnosis and Management of the Adult Psychiatric Patient in the Emergency Department." Annals of Emergency Medicine. Vol. 47. No. 1. Pages 79 to 99. January 2006.

- Maintain open posture (do not cross arms or clench fists).
- Coach patients on how to stay in control and clarify behavioral expectations.
- Verbalize respect and empathy.
- Position self at a 45° angle (directly in front of the patient can seem confrontational).
- Avoid sounding punitive or accusatory, as well as posturing to challenge.
- Give choices and encourage patient responsibility.
- Avoid confronting; rather, explore misconceptions.
- De-escalate security's show of force (if possible).[7]

If medication is deemed necessary for sedation, the ACEP clinical policy offers a recommendation for benzodiazepines or antipsychotics (**Table 2**).[5]

Involuntary Holds

Involuntary hospitalization occurs when the patient's risk to self or others, owing to mental illness, renders the hospitalization necessary to prevent harm.[6] Different jurisdictions have varied statutory approaches to how EPs go about holding patients. ACEP encourages EPs to be familiar with their state laws; however, there are some trends worth considering. For example, the duration of an emergency hold varies between 23 hours and 10 days (**Table 3**). Who can initiate a hold varies from any interested person to a guardian (**Table 4**). Reasons to hold can vary from danger to self to grave disability, including substance use disorder (**Table 5**). Furthermore, states vary with regard to judicial involvement before a hold (**Fig. 1**).

Warning and Protecting Third Parties

If a patient were to make a direct threat to harm another individual, then the EP has a duty to warn and protect that individual. Involuntary admission of the patient is sufficient to meet that duty to protect. If the patient is discharged and has made a clear and direct threat, then it is incumbent upon the EP to warn law enforcement. The landmark legal case in California of *Tarasoff v Regents of University of California* established California case law placing accountability on psychiatrists to prevent harm to third parties when a patient shares intention to harm them.[8] The 1974 decision regarding this case

Table 3
Duration of emergency holds and states' ability to extend holds without a court order

Duration	No Court Order Required	Court Order Required
23 h		ND
24 h		AZ, DE, IL, ME, MI, MT, NC, SC, UT
30 h		MD
48 h	GA, HI, IA	DC, TX
72 h	LA, NY, TN, VT, WA	AK, AR, CA, CO, CT, FL, IN, KY, MA, MN, MS, NJ, NV, OR, VA, WI, WY
96 h		MO, OH
5 d		ID, OK, PA, SD
7 d		AL, NM
10 d		NH, RI

Table 4
Who can initiate emergency commitment and judicial review requirements, by state

Initiator	No Requirement	Predetention Ex Parte Hearing	Postdetention Ex Parte Hearing
Any interested person	AZ, DE, LA, MA, MN, MO, NC, SD, UT, WV	AR, CO, MD, MS, VA, VT	IA, IN, ME, NH, TX
Relative	AZ, OK	MS, NY	NV
Friend	AZ		
Police officer	AL, CT, DE, FL, HI, LA, MA, MO, MT, OH, RI, WI	NY	KS, NV, TN, WY
Peace officer	AK, AZ, CA, CO, DE, IL, KY, LA, MD, MI, MT, NE, NM, OK, OR, PA, SD, TX, UT	NY	ME, MI, NH
Parole officer	OH		
Physician	AK, AZ, CT, DE, FL, GA, HI, KY, LA, MA, MD, MO, MN, NC, NJ, OH, OR, PA, RI, UT	NV	DC, ND, NH, NV, TN, WY
Nurse	AZ, MA, MO, NJ, RI	CO, FL, NY	ND
Advanced practice registered nurse	CT, GA, HI, LA, MD, MN		NH, WY
Physician assistant	HI, MN		WY
Psychologist	AK, CT, DE, GA, HI, LA, MA, MD, MN, MO, NC, NJ, OH, RI	FL, NY	DC, ND, NV, TN, WY
Psychiatrist	AK, AZ, DE, HI, MO, NJ, OH, RI, UT	VA	ND, NV, WY
Mental health professional	AL, CA, CO, DE, GA, HI, MA, MD, MN, MO, NE, RI, UT, WA	FL, KY	DC, ME, ND, NV, WY
Medical directors	CA, OR		
Hospital staff			ID
Attorney	HI	MS	
Judge	HI, IL, NJ	FL, VA	
Social worker	CT, GA, IL, HI, MA, MN, NJ, RI	CO, FL, NY	ND, NV, WY
Clergy	HI		
Government employee	DE, HI		
County-appointed professional	HI, MD, MS, PA		TN
Mental health program	MO, NJ		
Guardian	ID, OK	MS, NY	NV, TX

Reprinted with permission from Psychiatric Services, Volume 67, Issue 5, "State Laws on Emergency Holds for Mental Health Stabilization," Hedman et al., p. 530, p. 531, p. 532 (Copyright © 2016). American Psychiatric Association. All Rights Reserved.

Table 5
Reasons for emergency commitment, by state

State	Danger to Self	Danger to Others	Mentally Ill	Danger to Self due to Mental Illness	Danger to Others due to Mental Illness	Recently Attempted Suicide	Gravely Disabled	Unable to Meet Basic Needs
AK				✓	✓		✓	
AL				✓	✓			
AR	✓	✓						
AZ				✓	✓			
CA				✓	✓		✓	
CO				✓	✓		✓	
CT				✓	✓		✓	
DC				✓	✓			
DE				✓	✓			
FL				✓	✓			✓
GA			✓					
HI	✓	✓						
IA				✓	✓		✓	
ID				✓	✓		✓	
IL	✓	✓						
IN				✓	✓			
KS				✓	✓			✓
KY				✓	✓			
LA				✓	✓		✓	
MA				✓	✓			
MD	✓	✓						
ME				✓	✓			
MI				✓	✓			✓

State						
MN		✓		✓	✓	
MO	✓		✓	✓	✓	
MS				✓	✓	
MT	✓			✓	✓	
NC	✓		✓	✓	✓	
ND	✓			✓	✓	
NE				✓	✓	
NH	✓		✓	✓	✓	
NJ			✓	✓	✓	
NM			✓	✓	✓	
NV				✓	✓	
NY						✓ ✓
OH				✓	✓	
OK				✓	✓	
OR				✓	✓	
PA		✓	✓	✓	✓	
RI				✓	✓	
SC				✓	✓	
SD				✓	✓	
TN				✓	✓	
TX				✓	✓	
UT				✓	✓	
VA	✓			✓	✓	
VT				✓	✓	
WA	✓	✓		✓	✓	
WI				✓	✓	
WV				✓	✓	
WY				✓	✓	

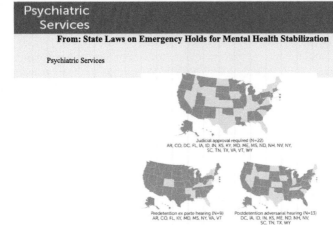

Fig. 1. State variation in requiring judicial approval before emergency holds. (Reprinted with permission from Psychiatric Services, Volume 67, Issue 5, "State Laws on Emergency Holds for Mental Health Stabilization," Hedman et al., p. 533 (Copyright © 2016). American Psychiatric Association. All Rights Reserved.)

codified a *duty to warn* third parties; however, the California Supreme Court's 1976 decision escalated this obligation to *duty to protect*.[9]

CASE 3

A 27-year-old nonbinary person presents to the ED complaining of anxiety. They state that they need to be admitted to the hospital. The psychiatry consultation service suspects malingering, as they have an outstanding warrant for arrest and are due to appear in court later this day. What should you do?

ESCAPING A TRIAL APPEARANCE

Patients presenting to the ED with anxiety or other mental health complaints may, in fact, be malingering. Most EPs are hesitant to make this diagnosis for fear of ignoring or dismissing a legitimate mental health concern. This is for good reason. One study found that ∼75% of patients diagnosed with malingering were found to have a psychiatric diagnosis other than malingering. Furthermore, these patients were found to more likely be men, over the age of 45, black, homeless, and high utilizers.[10] Concerns about justice in diagnosis are well-founded based on the demographics described. The *Diagnostic and Statistical Manual of Mental Disorders* (Fifth Edition) defines malingering as intentional production of false or grossly exaggerated physical or psychological symptoms, motivated by external incentives.[11] There are some pointed observations required before diagnosing malingering, including the following.

- Lack of cooperation during examination
- Historical evidence
- Exaggerated symptoms
- Evidence of antisocial personality disorder
- Conditional suicidality/homicidality
- Violence toward staff
- Under arrest/in police custody

SUMMARY

Patients presenting to the ED with mental health complaints deserve the same ethical treatment that would be afforded to the general population and typically require extra attention to concerns of autonomy, justice, and statutory frameworks. The voluntariness of suicidal patients is an important foundation for the approach to behavioral health treatment and should both be addressed by the EP early in the patient evaluation and nurtured even in the context of less-than-ideal patient boarding situations. When involuntary detainment is needed, solid understanding of local law and practice is needed to provide expedient psychiatric care. The authors recommend careful consideration of the context, timing, and motivation for patients presenting immediately before court appearances, but that patients' concerns should not be ignored out of hand, because pending legal action can be a valid trigger for mental health decompensation.

CLINICS CARE POINTS

- A familiarity with state laws surrounding involuntary holds will prepare you for more complicated ethical and legal dilemmas regarding involuntary detention for psychiatric reasons.
- Emergency physicians are well-qualified to medically screen patients complaining of mental health concerns and to lead efforts to de-escalate situations involving agitated patients.
- If malingering to avoid court appearance is identified, it can be directly addressed in the emergency department.

REFERENCES

1. Allen NG, Khan JS, Alzahri MS, Stolar AG. Ethical Issues in Emergency Psychiatry. Emerg Med Clin North Am. 2015;33(4):863–74.
2. Department of Health and Human Services. Health Information Portability and Accountability Act (HIPAA) Privacy Rule. 45 CFR 164.512. US.
3. Janlonski v. United States, 712 F. 2d 391 (9th Cir. 1983). case law.
4. Rajparia A. Ethical issues in emergency psychiatry. In: Maloy K, editor. A case-based approach to emergency psychiatry. New York: Oxford; 2016. p. 127–38.
5. Lukens TW, Wolf SJ, Edlow JA, et al. Clinical policy: critical issues in the diagnosis and management of the adult psychiatric patient in the emergency department. Ann Emerg Med 2006;47(1):79–99.
6. Cournos F, Faulkner L, Fitzgerald L, et al. Report of the task force on consent to voluntary hospitalization. Bull Am Acad Psychiatr Law 1993;21(3):293–307.
7. Hamm B. Ethical Practice in Emergency Psychiatry Common Dilemmas and Virtue-Informed Navigation. Psychiatr Clin 2021;44:627–40.
8. Fox PF. Commentary: So the pendulum swings – making sense of the duty to protect. J Am Acad Psychiatry Law 2010;38:474–8.
9. Tarasoff v. Regents of Univ. of Cal., 17 Cal. 3d 425, 131 Cal. Rptr. 14, 551 P.2d 334 (1976). California case law.
10. Park L, Costello S, Li J, et al. Race, health, and socioeconomic disparities associated with malingering in psychiatric patients at an urban emergency department. Gen Hosp Psychiatry 2021;71:121–7.
11. Diagnostic and statistical manual of mental disorders. 5th edition. Washington, DC: American Psychiatric Association; 2013.

Printed and bound by CPI Group (UK) Ltd, Croydon, CR0 4YY

08/05/2025

01864749-0003